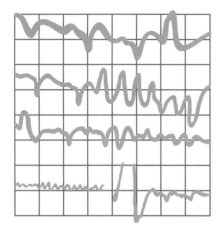

The
ECG
In Practice

SIXTH EDITION

John R. Hampton

DM MA DPhil FRCP FFPM FESC

Emeritus Professor of Cardiology,
University of Nottingham, UK

With contributions by

David Adlam BA BM BCh DPhil MRCP

Senior Lecturer in Acute and Interventional
Cardiology and Honorary Consultant
Cardiologist, University of Leicester, UK

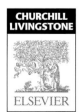

CHURCHILL
LIVINGSTONE

ELSEVIER

EDINBURGH LONDON NEW YORK OXFORD PHILADELPHIA ST LOUIS SYDNEY TORONTO 2013

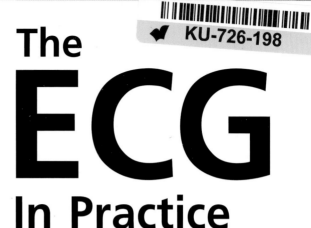

CHURCHILL LIVINGSTONE
ELSEVIER

© 2013 Elsevier Ltd. All rights reserved.

First edition 1986   Fourth edition 2003
Second edition 1992   Fifth edition 2008
Third edition 1997   Sixth edition 2013

ISBN 978-0-7020-4643-8
International ISBN 978-0-7020-4644-5
e-book ISBN 978-0-7020-5244-6

British Library Cataloguing in Publication Data
A catalogue record for this book is available from the British Library

Library of Congress Cataloging in Publication Data
A catalog record for this book is available from the Library of Congress

Notices

Knowledge and best practice in this field are constantly changing. As new research and experience broaden our understanding, changes in research methods, professional practices, or medical treatment may become necessary.

Practitioners and researchers must always rely on their own experience and knowledge in evaluating and using any information, methods, compounds, or experiments described herein. In using such information or methods they should be mindful of their own safety and the safety of others, including parties for whom they have a professional responsibility.

With respect to any drug or pharmaceutical products identified, readers are advised to check the most current information provided (i) on procedures featured or (ii) by the manufacturer of each product to be administered, to verify the recommended dose or formula, the method and duration of administration, and contraindications. It is the responsibility of practitioners, relying on their own experience and knowledge of their patients, to make diagnoses, to determine dosages and the best treatment for each individual patient, and to take all appropriate safety precautions.

To the fullest extent of the law, neither the publisher nor the authors, contributors, or editors, assume any liability for any injury and/or damage to persons or property as a matter of products liability, negligence or otherwise, or from any use or operation of any methods, products, instructions, or ideas contained in the material herein.

ELSEVIER your source for books, journals and multimedia in the health sciences

www.elsevierhealth.com

Working together to grow libraries in developing countries

www.elsevier.com • www.bookaid.org

The Publisher's policy is to use **paper manufactured from sustainable forests**

Printed in China

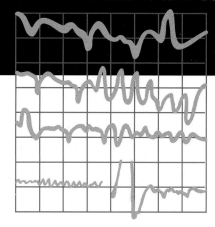

Preface

WHAT TO EXPECT OF THIS BOOK

I assume that the reader of this book will have the level of knowledge of the ECG that is contained in *The ECG Made Easy*, to which this is a companion volume. The ECG is indeed easy in principle, but the variations in pattern seen both in normal people and in patients with cardiac and other problems can make the ECG seem more complex than it really is. This book concentrates on these variations, and contains several examples of each abnormality. It is intended for anyone who understands the basics, but now wants to use the ECG to its maximum potential as a clinical tool.

The ECG is not an end in itself, but is an extension of the history and physical examination. Patients do not visit the doctor wanting an ECG, but come either for a health check or because they have symptoms. Therefore, this book is organized according to clinical situations, and the chapters cover the ECG in healthy subjects and in patients with palpitations, syncope, chest pain, breathlessness or non-cardiac conditions. To emphasize that the ECG is part of the general assessment of a patient, each chapter begins with a brief section on history and examination and ends with a short account of what might be done once the ECG has been interpreted.

This sixth edition continues the philosophy of its predecessors in that the patient is considered more important than the ECG. However, the ECG is a vital part of diagnosis and, increasingly, dictates treatment. Electrical devices of various sorts are standard treatment in cardiology, and patients with such devices are now commonly seen in patients who present with non-cardiological problems. Those who are not specialists in cardiology need to understand them. Therefore there is a series of changes in the text compared with previous editions, and the sections on pacemakers, defibrillators and electrophysiology have been integrated into the relevant chapters.

WHAT TO EXPECT OF THE ECG

The ECG has its limitations. Remember that it provides a picture of the electrical activity of the heart, but gives only an indirect indication of the heart's structure and function. It is, however, invaluable for assessing patients whose symptoms may be due to electrical malfunction in the heart, including patients with conduction problems and those with arrhythmias.

In healthy people, finding an apparently normal ECG may be reassuring. Unfortunately the ECG can be totally normal in patients with severe coronary disease. Conversely the range of normality is such that a healthy subject may quite wrongly be labelled as having heart disease on the basis of the ECG. Some ECG patterns that are undoubtedly abnormal (for example, right bundle branch block) are seen in perfectly healthy people. It is a good working principle that it is the individual's clinical state that matters, not the ECG.

When a patient complains of palpitations or syncope, the diagnosis of a cardiac cause is only certain if an ECG is recorded at the time of symptoms – but even when the patient is symptom-free, the ECG may provide a clue for the prepared mind. In patients with chest pain the ECG may indicate the diagnosis, and treatment can be based upon it, but it is essential to remember that the ECG may remain normal for a few hours after the onset of a myocardial infarction. In breathless patients a totally normal ECG probably rules out heart failure, but it is not a good way of diagnosing lung disease or pulmonary embolism. Finally, it must be remembered that the ECG can be quite abnormal in a patient with a variety of non-cardiac conditions, and one must not jump to the conclusion that an abnormal ECG indicates cardiac pathology.

ACKNOWLEDGEMENTS

In this sixth edition of *The ECG in Practice* I have been helped by many people. In particular, I am grateful to David Adlam for providing many illustrations, and for contributing the sections on devices and electrophysiology, which takes the book beyond the routine ECG into the realm of sophisticated diagnosis and electrical treatments – which are nevertheless based on an understanding of the ECG. I am also extremely grateful to my copy-editor, Alison Gale, for her enormous attention to detail that led to many improvements in the text. I am also grateful to Laurence Hunter and his team at Elsevier for their encouragement and patience. As before, I am grateful to many friends and colleagues who have helped me to find the wide range of examples of normal and abnormal ECGs that form the backbone of the book.

John Hampton
Nottingham, 2013

Contents

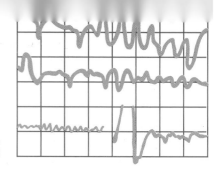

12-lead ECGs	viii
1. The ECG in healthy people	1
2. The ECG in patients with palpitations and syncope: between attacks	58
3. The ECG when the patient has a tachycardia	101
4. The ECG when the patient has a bradycardia	169
5. The ECG in patients with chest pain	208
6. The ECG in patients with breathlessness	287
7. The effect of other conditions on the ECG	316
8. Conclusions: four steps to making the most of the ECG	346
Index	350

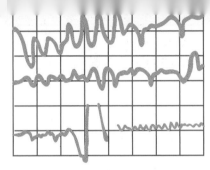

12-lead ECGs

AAI pacing 196
Accelerated idionodal rhythm 48
Accelerated idioventricular rhythm 28
Anorexia nervosa 342
Aortic stenosis, severe, left ventricular hypertrophy with 298
Aortic stenosis and left bundle branch block 296
Atrial fibrillation 124, 178
Atrial fibrillation, uncontrolled 290
Atrial fibrillation and anterior ischaemia 244
Atrial fibrillation and coupled ventricular extrasystoles 290
Atrial fibrillation and digoxin effect at rest 280
Atrial fibrillation and digoxin effect on exercise 280
Atrial fibrillation and inferior infarction 140
Atrial fibrillation and left bundle branch block 128, 130
Atrial fibrillation and right bundle branch block 134
Atrial fibrillation and Wolff–Parkinson-White syndrome 148

Atrial flutter and 1:1 conduction 120
Atrial flutter and 2:1 block 118
Atrial flutter and 4:1 block 120
Atrial flutter and intermittent VVI pacing 194
Atrial flutter and variable block 176
Atrial flutter in hypothermia 318
Atrial septal defect and right bundle branch block 326
Atrial tachycardia 110, 116
Atrioventricular nodal re-entry tachycardia (AVNRT) 122
Atrioventricular nodal re-entry tachycardia (AVNRT) and anterior ischaemia 244

Bifascicular block 90
Biventricular pacing 314
Broad complex tachycardia of uncertain origin 136, 138
Brugada syndrome 80

Chronic lung disease 310
Complete heart block 180

Complete heart block and Stokes–Adams attack 182
Congenital long QT syndrome 76

DDD pacing, atrial tracking 200
DDD pacing, atrial and ventricular pacing 198
DDD pacing, intermittent 200
Dextrocardia 10
Dextrocardia, leads reversed 10
Digoxin effect 334
Digoxin effect and ischaemia 262
Digoxin toxicity 336

Ebstein's anomaly, right atrial hypertrophy and right bundle branch block 324
Ectopic atrial rhythm 8
Electrical alternans 328
Exercise, digoxin effect, atrial fibrillation 280
Exercise-induced ischaemia 272
Exercise-induced ST segment depression 278
Exercise-induced ST segment elevation 274
Exercise testing, normal ECG 272, 278

Fallot's tetralogy, right ventricular hypertrophy in 324
Fascicular tachycardia 136
First degree block 84
First degree block and left bundle branch block 88
First degree block and right bundle branch block 90, 174, 182
Friedreich's ataxia 344

Hyperkalaemia 330
Hyperkalaemia, corrected 332
Hypertrophic cardiomyopathy 68, 300

Hypokalaemia 334
Hypothermia 318
Hypothermia, atrial flutter 318
Hypothermia, re-warming after 320

Intermittent VVI pacing 192
Ischaemia, anterior 242
Ischaemia, anterior and atrial fibrillation 244
Ischaemia, anterior and AV nodal re-entry tachycardia 244
Ischaemia, anterior and inferior infarction and right bundle branch block 238
Ischaemia, anterior and possible old inferior infarction 240
Ischaemia, anterior and right bundle branch block 238
Ischaemia, anterolateral 242
Ischaemia, digoxin effect and 262
Ischaemia, exercise-induced 272
Ischaemia, ?left ventricular hypertrophy 300
Ischaemia, probable 298

Junctional tachycardia with right bundle branch block 136

Left anterior hemiblock 88, 302
Left atrial hypertrophy 70
Left atrial hypertrophy and left ventricular hypertrophy 292
Left axis deviation 86
Left bundle branch block 66, 234
Left bundle branch block and aortic stenosis 296
Left bundle branch block and ?right ventricular overload 234
Left posterior hemiblock 92
Left ventricular hypertrophy 64, 252, 260, 294,

296, 322
Left ventricular hypertrophy and ?ischaemia 300
Left ventricular hypertrophy and left atrial hypertrophy 292
Left ventricular hypertrophy and severe aortic stenosis 298
Lithium treatment 340
Long QT syndrome, congenital 76
Long QT syndrome, drug toxicity 146
Lown–Ganong–Levine syndrome 74

Malignant pericardial effusion 328
Mediastinal shift 22
Mitral stenosis and pulmonary hypertension 292
Myocardial infarction, acute anterior and old inferior 232
Myocardial infarction, acute anterolateral, with left axis deviation 222
Myocardial infarction, acute inferior 214
Myocardial infarction, acute inferior and anterior ischaemia 230
Myocardial infarction, acute inferior (STEMI) and anterior NSTEMI 232
Myocardial infarction, acute inferior and old anterior 230
Myocardial infarction, acute inferior and RBBB 236
Myocardial infarction, acute lateral 220
Myocardial infarction, anterior 218
Myocardial infarction, anterior, ?age 274
Myocardial infarction, anterior NSTEMI 240
Myocardial infarction, anterolateral, ?age 224
Myocardial infarction, evolving inferior 216
Myocardial infarction, inferior and atrial fibrillation 140
Myocardial infarction, inferior and right bundle branch block 236

Myocardial infarction, inferior and right bundle branch block and ?anterior ischaemia 238
Myocardial infarction, inferior and right ventricular infarction 228
Myocardial infarction, inferior and ventricular tachycardia 140
Myocardial infarction, lateral (after 3 days) 222
Myocardial infarction, old anterior 224
Myocardial infarction, old anterolateral NSTEMI 260
Myocardial infarction, old inferior (possible) and anterior ischaemia 240
Myocardial infarction, old posterior 254
Myocardial infarction, posterior 226
Myocardial infarction, posterior infarct with normal QT interval 78

Normal ECG 8, 12, 272, 278
Normal ECG, accelerated idionodal rhythm 48
Normal ECG, black people 42
Normal ECG, child 52
Normal ECG, ectopic atrial rhythm 8
Normal ECG, exercise testing 272, 278
Normal ECG, high take-off ST segment 32
Normal ECG, junctional escape beat 4
Normal ECG, left axis deviation 50
Normal ECG, 'leftward' limit of normality 16
Normal ECG, notched (bifid) P wave 12
Normal ECG, notched S wave (V_2) 26
Normal ECG, P wave, bifid (notched) 12
Normal ECG, P wave inversion 8, 40
Normal ECG, P wave inversion (lead VR, VL) 40
Normal ECG, partial right bundle branch block pattern 34
Normal ECG, PR interval variation 48
Normal ECG, pre-exercise 282

Normal ECG, R wave, tall (voltage criteria and) 294
Normal ECG, R wave dominance (lead II) 14
Normal ECG, R wave dominance (V_1) 22, 308
Normal ECG, R wave dominance (V_3) 20
Normal ECG, R wave dominance (V_4) 18
Normal ECG, R wave dominance (V_5) 20, 24
Normal ECG, R wave dominance (V_6) 18
Normal ECG, R wave size 14
Normal ECG, right axis deviation 16
Normal ECG, 'rightward' limit of normality 14
Normal ECG, R–R interval variation 2
Normal ECG, RSR[1] pattern 26
Normal ECG, RSR[1]S[1] pattern 26
Normal ECG, S wave dominance (lead I) 16
Normal ECG, S wave dominance (lead III) 16
Normal ECG, S wave dominance (V_1) 18
Normal ECG, S wave dominance (V_2) 20, 24
Normal ECG, S wave dominance (V_3) 18
Normal ECG, S wave dominance (V_4) 20
Normal ECG, septal Q wave 28, 50
Normal ECG, small Q wave 30, 38
Normal ECG, ST segment, isoelectric and sloping upward 30
Normal ECG, ST segment depression 34
Normal ECG, ST segment depression (nonspecific) 36
Normal ECG, ST segment elevation 32
Normal ECG, T wave, biphasic 34, 40, 52
Normal ECG, T wave, peaked 332
Normal ECG, T wave, tall peaked 44
Normal ECG, T wave flattening 44
Normal ECG, T wave inversion (lead III) 38
Normal ECG, T wave inversion (lead V_1) 38
Normal ECG, T wave inversion (lead V_2) 40
Normal ECG, T wave inversion (lead V_3) 42
Normal ECG, T wave inversion (lead VR) 36

Normal ECG, T wave inversion (lead VR, V_1–V_2) 40
Normal ECG, T wave inversion (lead VR, VL) 40, 42
Normal ECG, T wave inversion in black people 42
Normal ECG, U wave, prominent/large 46, 50

Pericardial effusion, malignant 328
Pericarditis 250
Pre-exercise normal ECG 282
Prolonged QT interval due to amiodarone 78, 338
Pseudonormalization 276
Pulmonary embolus 246, 248, 250, 310
Pulmonary hypertension and mitral stenosis 292
Pulmonary stenosis 322

Re-warming after hypothermia 320
Right atrial hypertrophy 304
Right atrial hypertrophy and right bundle branch block, in Ebstein's anomaly 324
Right atrial hypertrophy and right ventricular hypertrophy 304
Right bundle branch block and acute inferior infarction 236
Right bundle branch block and anterior infarction 236
Right bundle branch block and anterior ischaemia 238
Right bundle branch block and atrial septal defect 326
Right bundle branch block and inferior infarction, ?anterior ischaemia 238
Right bundle branch block and right atrial hypertrophy, in Ebstein's anomaly 324
Right ventricular hypertrophy 66, 308
Right ventricular hypertrophy, marked 306
Right ventricular hypertrophy in Fallot's tetralogy 324

Right ventricular hypertrophy and right atrial hypertrophy 304
Right ventricular outflow tract ventricular tachycardia (RVOT-VT) 104, 144
RSR^1 pattern 26, 80
RSR^{1}S^1 pattern 26

Second degree block (2:1) 86, 180
Second degree block (Wenckebach) 84
Second degree block and left anterior hemiblock 94
Second degree block and left anterior hemiblock and right bundle branch block 94
Sick sinus syndrome 172
Sinus arrhythmia 2, 112
Sinus bradycardia 4, 170, 172
Sinus rhythm, after cardioversion 118, 122, 138
Sinus rhythm, in Wolff–Parkinson-White syndrome type A 108
Sinus rhythm and left bundle branch block 128
Sinus rhythm and normal conduction, post-cardioversion 138
Sinus tachycardia 4, 112
ST segment, nonspecific changes 210
ST segment depression, exercise-induced 278
ST segment elevation, exercise-induced 274
Subarachnoid haemorrhage 344
Supraventricular extrasystole 6, 114

Supraventricular tachycardia 106

T wave, nonspecific changes 210
T wave, nonspecific flattening 262
T wave, unexplained abnormality 258
Thyrotoxicosis 326
Trauma 342
Trifascicular block 92

Ventricular extrasystole 6, 114
Ventricular extrasystoles, coupled and atrial fibrillation 290
Ventricular fibrillation 162
Ventricular tachycardia 132, 134
Ventricular tachycardia, fusion and capture beats 142
Ventricular tachycardia and inferior infarction 140
VVI pacing, bipolar 190
VVI pacing, intermittent 192
VVI pacing, unipolar 192
VVI pacing in complete block 194

Wolff–Parkinson-White syndrome and atrial fibrillation 148
Wolff–Parkinson-White syndrome type A 70, 72, 148, 256, 302
Wolff–Parkinson-White syndrome type B 74, 258

The ECG in healthy people

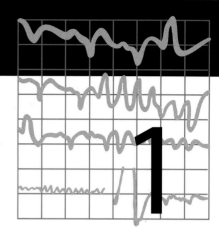

The 'normal' ECG	**2**
The normal cardiac rhythm	2
The heart rate	2
Extrasystoles	7
The P wave	7
The PR interval	13
The QRS complex	15
The ST segment	31
The T wave	37
The QT interval	48
The ECG in athletes	48
The ECG in pregnancy	52
The ECG in children	52
Frequency of ECG abnormalities in healthy people	54

What to do	**54**
The range of normality	54
The prognosis of patients with an abnormal ECG	54
Further investigations	56
Treatment of asymptomatic ECG abnormalities	56

For the purposes of this chapter, we shall assume that the subject from whom the ECG was recorded is asymptomatic, and that physical examination has revealed no abnormalities. We need to consider the range of normality of the ECG, but of course we cannot escape from the fact that not all disease causes symptoms or abnormal signs, and a subject who appears healthy may not be so and may therefore have an abnormal ECG. In particular, individuals who present for screening may well have symptoms about which they have not consulted a doctor, so it cannot

1

be assumed that an ECG obtained through a screening programme has come from a healthy subject.

The range of normality in the ECG is therefore debatable. We first have to consider the variations in the ECG that we can expect to find in completely healthy people, and then we can think about the significance of ECGs that are undoubtedly 'abnormal'.

THE 'NORMAL' ECG

THE NORMAL CARDIAC RHYTHM

Sinus rhythm is the only normal sustained rhythm. In young people the R–R interval is reduced (i.e. the heart rate is increased) during inspiration, and this is called sinus arrhythmia (Fig. 1.1). When sinus arrhythmia is marked, it may mimic an atrial arrhythmia. However, in sinus arrhythmia each P–QRS–T complex is normal, and it is only the interval between them that changes.

Sinus arrhythmia becomes less marked with increasing age of the subject, and is lost in conditions such as diabetic autonomic neuropathy due to impairment of the vagus nerve function.

THE HEART RATE

There is no such thing as a normal heart rate, and the terms 'tachycardia' and 'bradycardia' should be used

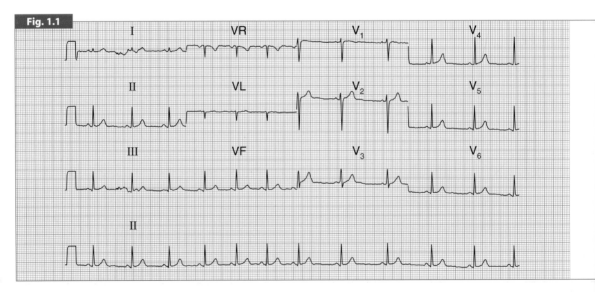

Fig. 1.1

with care. There is no point at which a high heart rate in sinus rhythm has to be called 'sinus tachycardia' and there is no upper limit for 'sinus bradycardia'. Nevertheless, unexpectedly fast or slow rates do need an explanation.

SINUS TACHYCARDIA

The ECG in Figure 1.2 was recorded from a young woman who complained of a fast heart rate. She had no other symptoms, but was anxious. There were no other abnormalities on examination, and her blood count and thyroid function tests were normal.

Box 1.1 shows possible causes of sinus rhythm with a fast heart rate.

Box 1.1 Possible causes of sinus rhythm with a fast heart rate

- Pain, fright, exercise
- Hypovolaemia
- Myocardial infarction
- Heart failure
- Pulmonary embolism
- Obesity
- Lack of physical fitness
- Pregnancy
- Thyrotoxicosis
- Anaemia
- Beri-beri
- CO_2 retention
- Autonomic neuropathy
- Drugs:
  - sympathomimetics
  - salbutamol (including by inhalation)
  - caffeine
  - atropine

Sinus arrhythmia

Note
- Marked variation in R–R interval
- Constant PR interval
- Constant shape of P wave and QRS complex

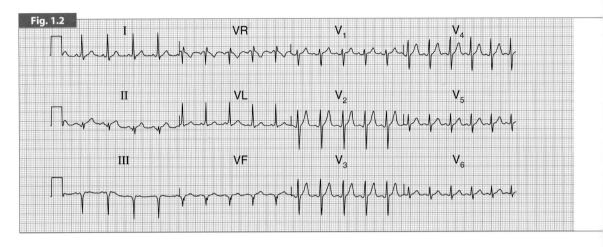

Fig. 1.2

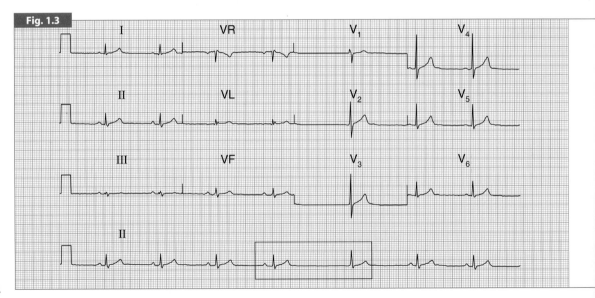

Fig. 1.3

4

Sinus tachycardia

Note
- Normal P–QRS–T waves
- R–R interval 500 ms
- Heart rate 120/min

SINUS BRADYCARDIA

The ECG in Figure 1.3 was recorded from a young professional footballer. His heart rate was 44/min, and at one point the sinus rate became so slow that a junctional escape beat appeared.

The possible causes of sinus rhythm with a slow heart rate are summarized in Box 1.2.

Sinus bradycardia

Note
- Sinus rhythm
- Rate 44/min
- One junctional escape beat

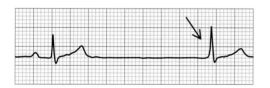

Junctional escape beat

Box 1.2 Possible causes of sinus rhythm with a slow heart rate

- Physical fitness
- Vasovagal attacks
- Sick sinus syndrome
- Acute myocardial infarction, especially inferior
- Hypothyroidism
- Hypothermia
- Obstructive jaundice
- Raised intracranial pressure
- Drugs:
  - beta-blockers (including eye drops for glaucoma)
  - verapamil
  - digoxin

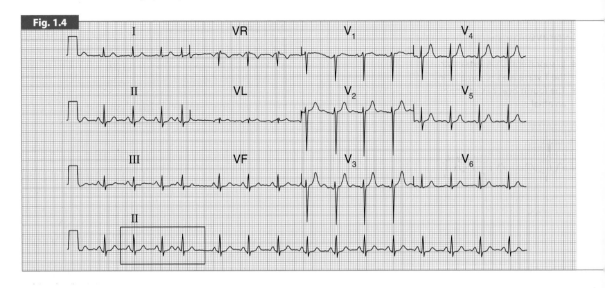

Fig. 1.4

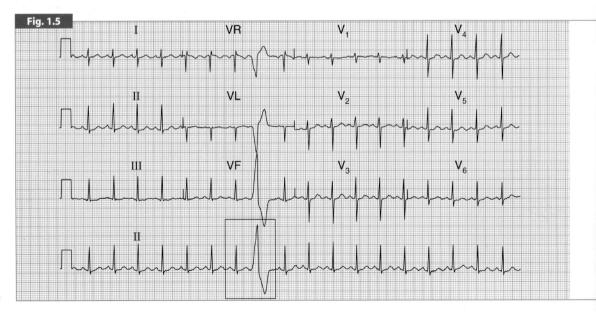

Fig. 1.5

Supraventricular extrasystole
Note
- In supraventricular extrasystoles the QRS complex and the T wave are the same as in the sinus beat
- The fourth beat has an abnormal P wave and therefore an atrial origin

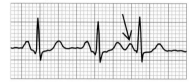

Early abnormal P wave

Ventricular extrasystole
Note
- Sinus rhythm, with one ventricular extrasystole
- Extrasystole has a wide and abnormal QRS complex and an abnormal T wave

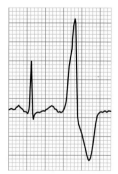

Ventricular extrasystole

EXTRASYSTOLES

Supraventricular extrasystoles, either atrial or junctional (AV nodal), occur commonly in normal people and are of no significance. Atrial extrasystoles (Fig. 1.4) have an abnormal P wave; in junctional extrasystoles either there is no P wave or the P wave may follow the QRS complex.

Ventricular extrasystoles are also commonly seen in normal ECGs (Fig. 1.5).

In healthy people, normal sinus rhythm may be replaced by what are, in effect, repeated atrial extrasystoles. This is sometimes called an 'ectopic atrial rhythm' and it is of no particular significance (Fig. 1.6).

THE P WAVE

In sinus rhythm, the P wave is normally upright in all leads except VR. When the QRS complex is predominantly downward in lead VL, the P wave may also be inverted (Fig. 1.7).

In patients with dextrocardia the P wave is inverted in lead I (Fig. 1.8). In practice this is more often seen if the limb leads have been wrongly attached, but dextrocardia can be recognized if leads V_5 and V_6, which normally 'look at' the left ventricle, show a predominantly downward QRS complex.

If the ECG of a patient with dextrocardia is repeated with the limb leads reversed, and the chest leads are placed on the right side of the chest instead of the left, in corresponding positions, the ECG becomes like that of a normal patient (Fig. 1.9).

A notched or bifid P wave is the hallmark of left atrial hypertrophy, and peaked P waves indicate right atrial hypertrophy – but bifid or peaked P waves can also be seen with normal hearts (Fig. 1.10).

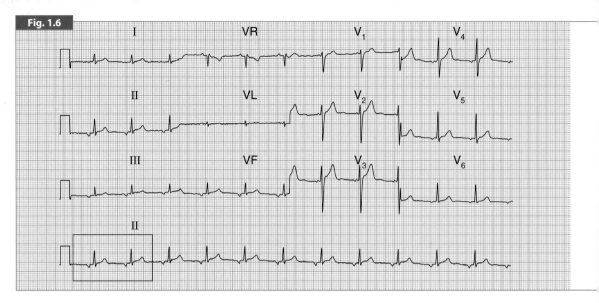

Fig. 1.6

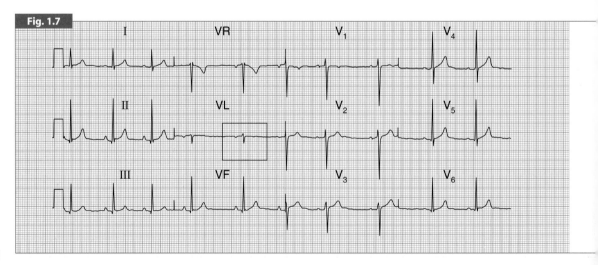

Fig. 1.7

Normal variant: ectopic atrial rhythm

Note
- Sinus rhythm
- Inverted P wave in leads II–III, VF, V_4–V_6
- Constant PR interval

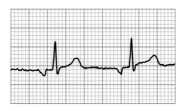

Inverted P waves in lead II

Normal ECG

Note
- In both leads VR and VL the P wave is inverted, and the QRS complex is predominantly downward

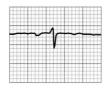

Inverted P wave in lead VL

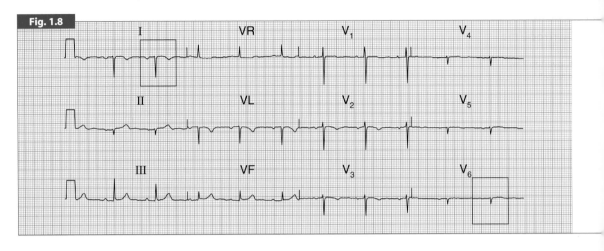

Fig. 1.8

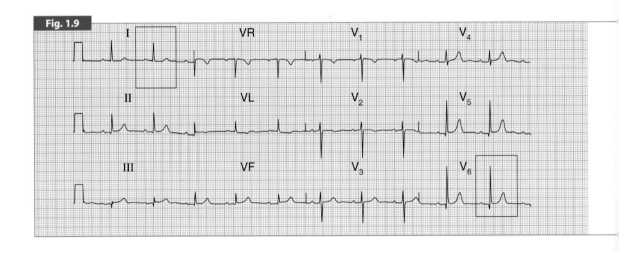

Fig. 1.9

Dextrocardia

Note
- Inverted P wave in lead I
- No left ventricular complexes seen in leads V_5–V_6

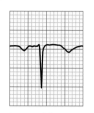 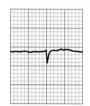

Inverted P wave
and dominant S
wave in lead I

Persistent S wave
in lead V_6

Dextrocardia, leads reversed

Note
- Same patient as in Figure 1.8
- P wave in lead I upright
- QRS complex upright in lead I
- Typical left ventricular complex in lead V_6

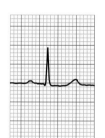 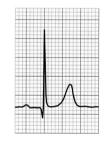

Upright P wave and
QRS complex in lead I

Normal QRS complex
in lead V_6

Fig. 1.10

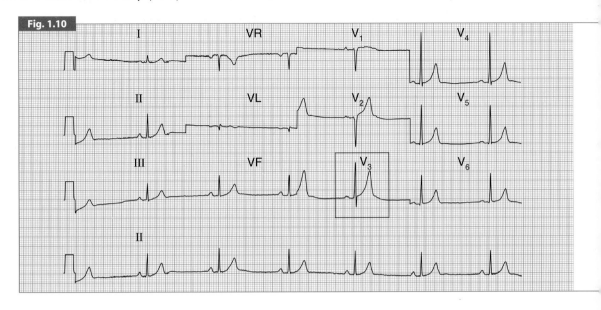

Fig. 1.11

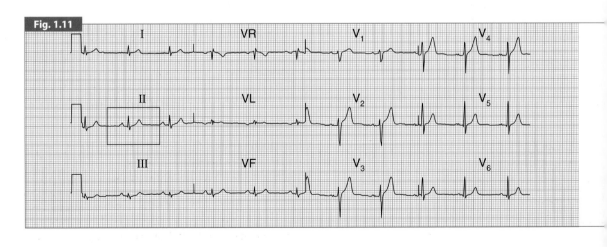

Normal ECG

Note

- Sinus rhythm
- Bifid P waves, best seen in leads V_2–V_4
- Peaked T waves and U waves, best seen in leads V_2–V_3 – normal variants

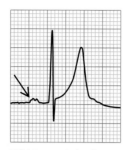

Bifid P wave in lead V_3

Normal ECG

Note

- PR interval 170 ms
- PR interval constant in all leads
- Notched P wave in lead V_5 is often normal

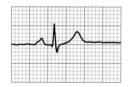

PR interval 170 ms

THE PR INTERVAL

In sinus rhythm, the PR interval is constant and its normal range is 120–200 ms (3–5 small squares of ECG paper) (Fig. 1.11). In atrial extrasystoles, or ectopic atrial rhythms, the PR interval may be short, and a PR interval of less than 120 ms suggests pre-excitation.

A PR interval of longer than 220 ms may be due to first degree block, but the ECGs of healthy individuals, especially athletes, may have PR intervals of slightly longer than 220 ms – which can be ignored in the absence of any other indication of heart disease.

PR interval 'abnormalities' will be discussed further in the context of normal people in Chapter 2.

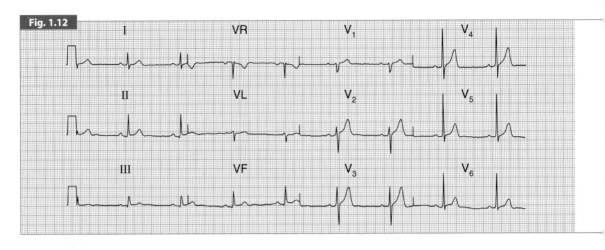

Fig. 1.12

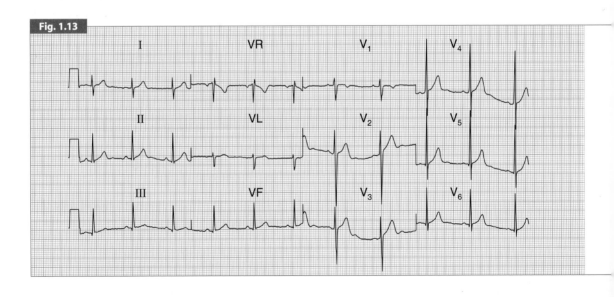

Fig. 1.13

Normal ECG
Note
- QRS complex upright in leads I–III
- R wave tallest in lead II

Normal ECG
Note
- This record shows the 'rightward' limit of normality of the cardiac axis
- R and S waves equal in lead I

THE QRS COMPLEX

THE CARDIAC AXIS

There is a fairly wide range of normality in the direction of the cardiac axis. In most people the QRS complex is tallest in lead II, but in leads I and III the QRS complex is also predominantly upright (i.e. the R wave is greater than the S wave) (Fig. 1.12).

The cardiac axis is still perfectly normal when the R wave and S wave are equal in lead I: this is common in tall people (Fig. 1.13).

When the S wave is greater than the R wave in lead I, right axis deviation is present. However, this is very common in perfectly normal people. The ECG in Figure 1.14 is from a professional footballer.

It is common for the S wave to be greater than the R wave in lead III, and the cardiac axis can still be considered normal when the S wave equals the R wave in lead II (Fig. 1.15). These patterns are common in fat people and during pregnancy.

When the depth of the S wave exceeds the height of the R wave in lead II, left axis deviation is present (see Figs 2.25 and 2.26).

Fig. 1.14

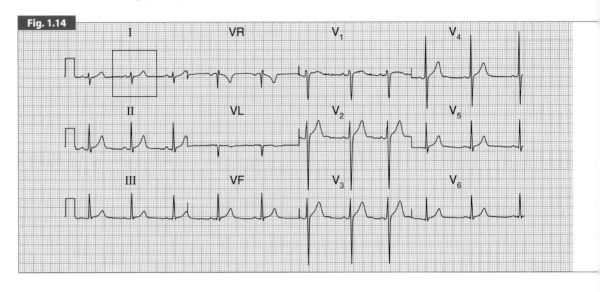

Fig. 1.15

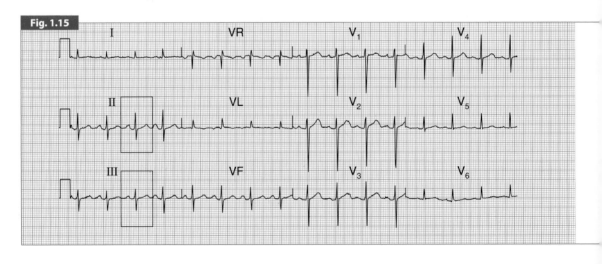

?Normal ECG

Note
- Right axis deviation: S wave greater than R wave in lead I
- Upright QRS complexes in leads II–III

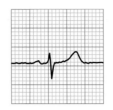

Dominant S wave in lead I

Normal ECG

Note
- This shows the 'leftward' limit of normality of the cardiac axis
- S wave equals R wave in lead II
- S wave greater than R wave in lead III

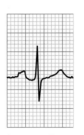 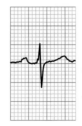

S wave = R   S wave > R
wave in lead II   wave in lead III

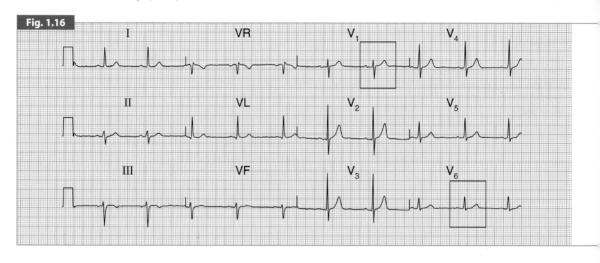

Fig. 1.16

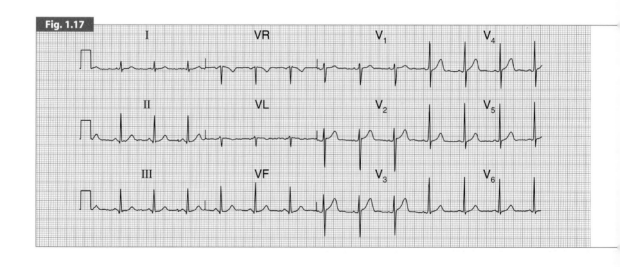

Fig. 1.17

Normal ECG

Note

- Lead V_1 shows a predominantly downward complex, with the S wave greater than the R wave
- Lead V_6 shows an upright complex, with a dominant R wave and a tiny S wave

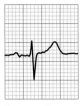 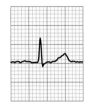

S wave > R
wave in lead V_1

Dominant R
wave in lead V_6

Normal ECG

Note

- In lead V_3 there is a dominant S wave
- In lead V_4 there is a dominant R wave
- The transition point is between leads V_3 and V_4

THE SIZE OF R AND S WAVES IN THE CHEST LEADS

In lead V_1 there should be a small R wave and a deep S wave, and the balance between the two should change progressively from V_1 to V_6. In lead V_6 there should be a tall R wave and no S wave (Fig. 1.16).

Typically the 'transition point', when the R and S waves are equal, is seen in lead V_3 or V_4 but there is quite a lot of variation. Figure 1.17 shows an ECG in which the transition point is somewhere between leads V_3 and V_4.

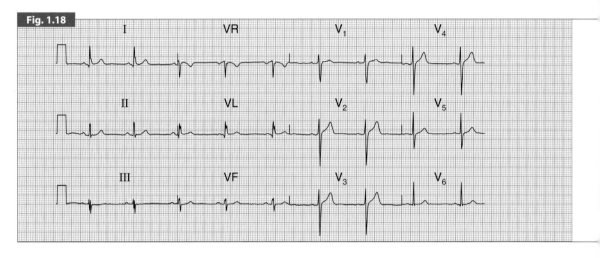

Fig. 1.18

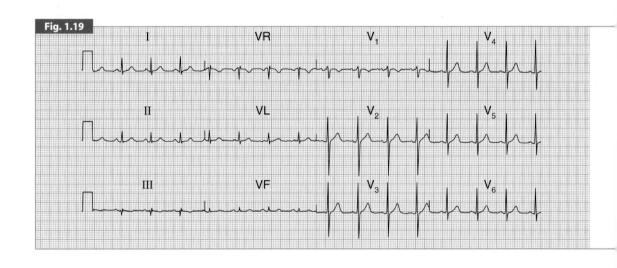

Fig. 1.19

Normal ECG

Note

- Dominant S wave in lead V_4
- R wave just bigger than S wave in lead V_5

Normal ECG

Note

- Dominant S wave in lead V_2
- Dominant R wave in lead V_3
- The transition point is between leads V_2 and V_3

Figure 1.18 shows an ECG with a transition point between leads V_4 and V_5, and Figure 1.19 shows an ECG with a transition point between leads V_2 and V_3.

The transition point is typically seen in lead V_5 or even V_6 in patients with chronic lung disease (see Ch. 6), and this is called 'clockwise rotation'. In extreme cases, the chest lead needs to be placed in the posterior axillary line, or even further round to the back (leads V_7–V_9) before the transition point is demonstrated. A similar ECG pattern may be seen in patients with an abnormal chest shape, particularly when depression of the sternum shifts the mediastinum to the left, although in this case the term 'clockwise rotation' is not used. The patient from whom the ECG in Figure 1.20 was recorded had mediastinal shift.

Occasionally the ECG of a totally normal subject will show a 'dominant' R wave (i.e. the height of the R wave exceeds the depth of the S wave) in lead V_1. There will thus, effectively, be no transition point, and this is called 'counterclockwise rotation'. The ECG in Figure 1.21 was recorded from a healthy footballer with a normal heart. However, a dominant R wave in lead V_1 is usually due to either right ventricular hypertrophy (see Ch. 6) or a true posterior infarction (see Ch. 5).

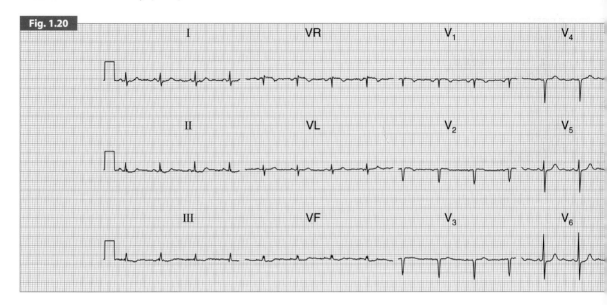

Fig. 1.20

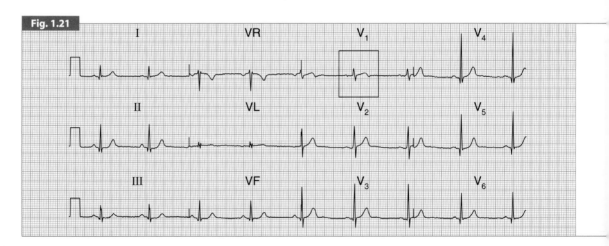

Fig. 1.21

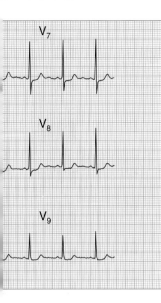

Mediastinal shift
Note
- 'Abnormal' ECG, but a normal heart
- Shift of the mediastinum means that the transition point is under lead V_6
- Ventricular complexes are shown in leads round the left side of the chest, in positions V_7–V_9

Normal ECG
Note
- Dominant R waves in lead V_1

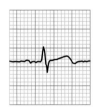

Dominant R wave in lead V_1

23

Fig. 1.22

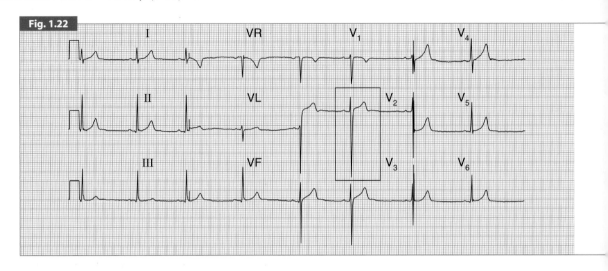

Fig. 1.23

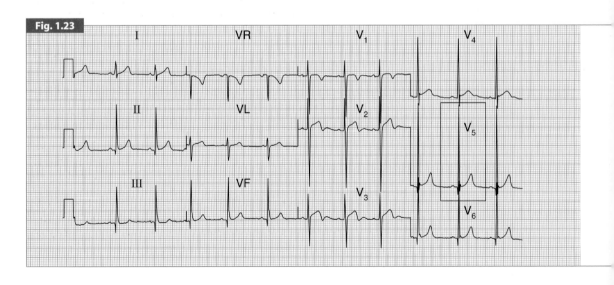

Normal ECG

Note
- S wave in lead V_2 is 36 mm

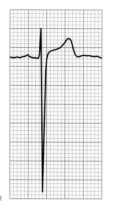

S wave > 25 mm in lead V_2

Normal ECG

Note
- R wave in lead V_5 is 42 mm

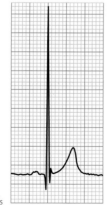

R wave > 25 mm in lead V_5

Although the balance between the height of the R wave and the depth of the S wave is significant for the identification of cardiac axis deviation, or right ventricular hypertrophy, the absolute height of the R wave provides little useful information. Provided that the ECG is properly calibrated (1 mV causes 1 cm of vertical deflection on the ECG), the limits for the sizes of the R and S waves in normal subjects are usually said to be:

- 25 mm for the R wave in lead V_5 or V_6
- 25 mm for the S wave in lead V_1 or V_2
- Sum of R wave in lead V_5 or V_6 plus S wave in lead V_1 or V_2 should be less than 35 mm.

However, R waves taller than 25 mm are commonly seen in leads V_5–V_6 in fit and thin young people, and are perfectly normal. Thus, these 'limits' are not helpful. The ECGs in Figures 1.22 and 1.23 were both recorded from fit young men with normal hearts.

THE WIDTH OF THE QRS COMPLEX

The QRS complex should be less than 120 ms in duration (i.e. less than 3 small squares) in all leads. If it is longer than this, then either the ventricles have been depolarized from a ventricular rather than a supraventricular focus (i.e. a ventricular rhythm is present), or there is an abnormality of conduction within the ventricles. The latter is most commonly due to bundle branch block. An RSR[1] pattern, resembling that of right bundle branch block but with a narrow QRS complex, is sometimes called 'partial right bundle branch block' and is a normal variant (Fig. 1.24). An RSR[1]S[1] pattern is also a normal variant (Fig. 1.25), and is sometimes called a 'splintered' complex.

Fig. 1.24

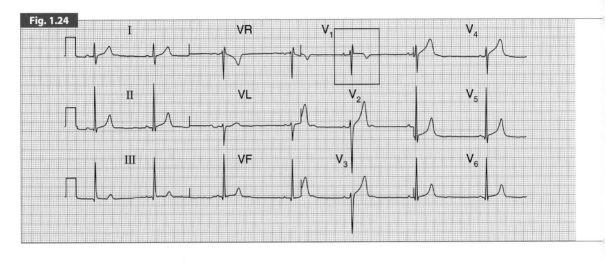

Fig. 1.25

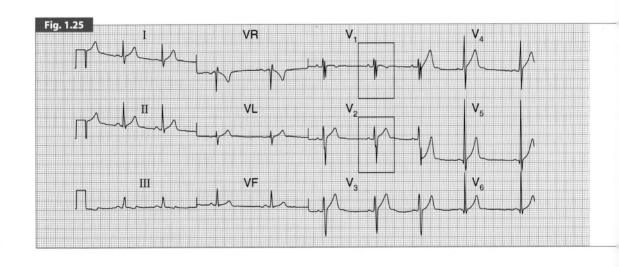

Normal ECG
Note
- RSR¹ pattern in lead V_2
- QRS complex duration 100 ms
- Partial right bundle branch block pattern

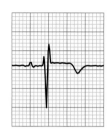

RSR¹ pattern and QRS complex 100 ms in lead V_1

Normal ECG
Note
- RSR¹S¹ pattern in lead V_1
- Notched S wave in lead V_2
- QRS complex duration 100 ms
- Partial right bundle branch block pattern

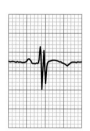 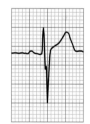

RSR¹S¹ pattern in lead V_1

Notched S wave in lead V_2

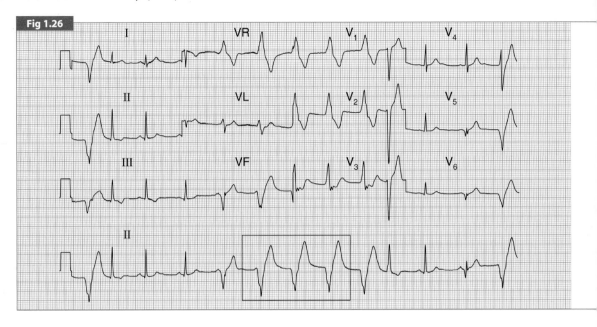

Fig 1.26

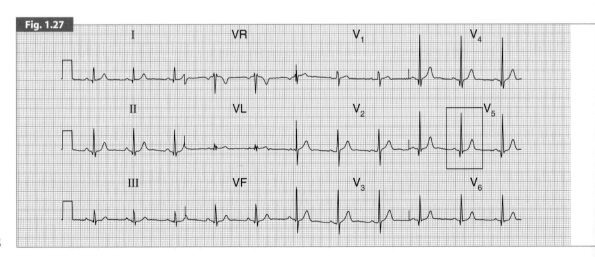

Fig. 1.27

Accelerated idioventricular rhythm

Note
- Sinus rhythm
- First and last beats are ventricular extrasystoles
- The fifth beat starts a run of ventricular rhythm at about 80/min

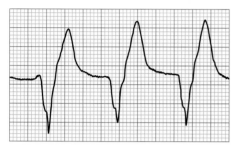

Idioventricular rhythm in lead II

In perfectly normal hearts the normal rhythm may be replaced by an accelerated idioventricular rhythm, which looks like a run of regular ventricular extrasystoles, with wide QRS complexes (Fig. 1.26).

Q WAVES

The normal depolarization of the interventricular septum from left to right causes a small 'septal' Q wave in any of leads II, VL or V_5–V_6. Septal Q waves are usually less than 3 mm deep and less than 1 mm across (Fig. 1.27).

A small Q wave is also common in lead III in normal people, in which case it is always narrow but can be more than 3 mm deep. Occasionally there will be a similar Q wave in lead VF (Fig. 1.28). These 'normal' Q waves become much less deep, and may disappear altogether, on deep inspiration (see Fig. 1.36).

Normal ECG

Note
- Septal Q waves in leads I, II, V_4–V_6

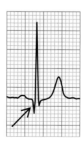

Septal Q wave in lead V_5

29

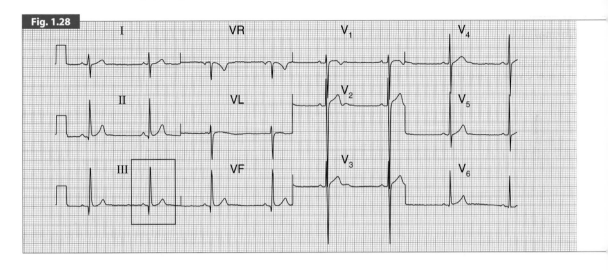

Fig. 1.28

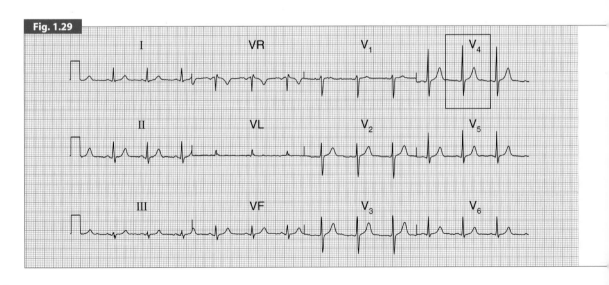

Fig. 1.29

Normal ECG

Note

- Narrow but quite deep Q wave in lead III
- Smaller Q wave in lead VF

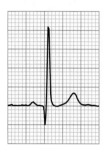

Narrow Q wave in lead III

Normal ECG

Note

- ST segment is isoelectric but slopes upwards in leads V_2–V_5

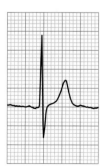

Upward-sloping ST segment in lead V_4

THE ST SEGMENT

The ST segment (the part of the ECG between the S wave and the T wave) should be horizontal and 'iso-electric', which means that it should be at the same level as the baseline of the record between the end of the T wave and the next P wave. However, in the chest leads the ST segment often slopes upwards and is not easy to define (Fig. 1.29).

An elevation of the ST segment is the hallmark of an acute myocardial infarction (see Ch. 5), and depression of the ST segment can indicate ischaemia or the effect of digoxin. However, it is perfectly normal for the ST segment to be elevated following an S wave in leads V_2–V_5. This is sometimes called a 'high take-off ST segment'. The ECGs in Figures 1.30 and 1.31 were recorded from perfectly healthy young men.

The ST segment is apparently raised when there is 'early repolarization', which causes the ST segment to be arched, and is usually only seen in the anterior leads, not the limb leads (see Fig. 1.39).

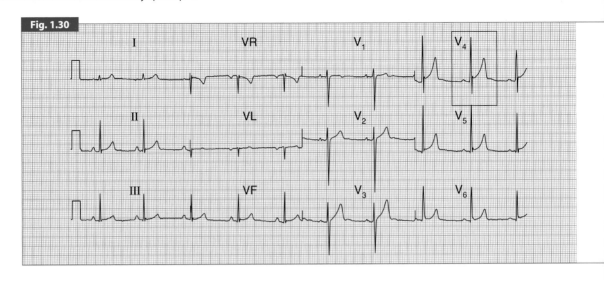

Fig. 1.30

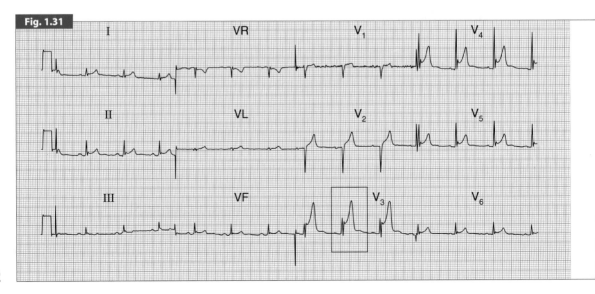

Fig. 1.31

Normal ECG
Note
- In lead V$_4$ there is an S wave followed by a raised ST segment. This is a 'high take-off' ST segment

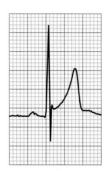

High take-off ST segment in lead V$_4$

Normal ECG
Note
- Marked ST segment elevation in lead V$_3$ follows an S wave

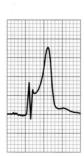

High take-off ST segment in lead V$_3$

Box 1.3 shows the possible causes of ST segment elevation, other than myocardial infarction.

ST segment depression is measured relative to the baseline (between the T and P waves), 60–80 ms after the 'J' point, which is the point of inflection at the junction of the S wave and the ST segment. Minor depression of the ST segment is not uncommon in normal people, and is then called 'nonspecific'; the advantage of using this word is that it leaves the way open for a later change of diagnosis. ST segment depression in lead III but not VF is likely to be nonspecific (Fig. 1.32). Nonspecific ST segment depression should not be more than 2 mm (Fig. 1.33), and the segment often slopes upwards. Horizontal ST segment depression of more than 2 mm indicates ischaemia (see Ch. 5).

Fig. 1.32

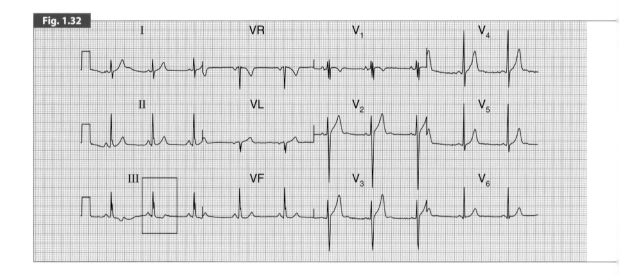

Box 1.3 Causes of ST segment elevation other than myocardial infarction

- Normal variants (high take-off and early repolarization)
- Left bundle branch block
- Acute pericarditis and myocarditis
- Hyperkalaemia
- Brugada syndrome
- Arrhythmogenic right ventricular cardiomyopathy
- Pulmonary embolism

Normal ECG

Note
- ST segment depression in lead III but not VF
- Biphasic T wave (i.e. initially inverted but then upright) in lead III but not VF
- Partial right bundle branch block pattern

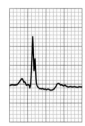

ST segment depression and biphasic T wave in lead III

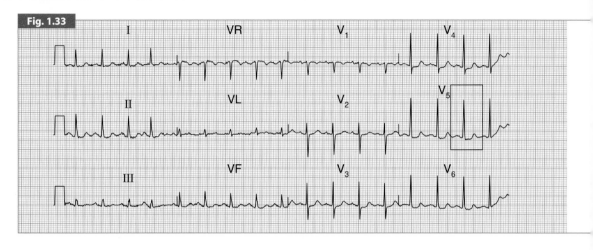

Fig. 1.33

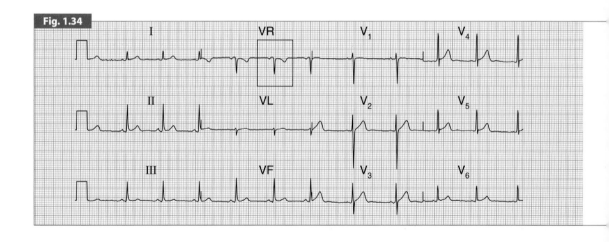

Fig. 1.34

Possibly normal ECG

Note

- ST segment depression of 1 mm in leads V_3–V_6
- In a patient with chest pain this would raise suspicions of ischaemia but, particularly in women, such changes can be nonspecific

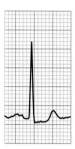

Nonspecific ST segment depression in lead V_5

Normal ECG

Note

- T wave is inverted in lead VR but is upright in all other leads

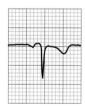

Inverted T wave in lead VR

THE T WAVE

In a normal ECG the T wave is always inverted in lead VR, and often in lead V_1, but is usually upright in all the other leads (Fig. 1.34).

The T wave is also often inverted in lead III but not VF. However, its inversion in lead III may be reversed on deep inspiration (Figs 1.35 and 1.36).

Fig. 1.35

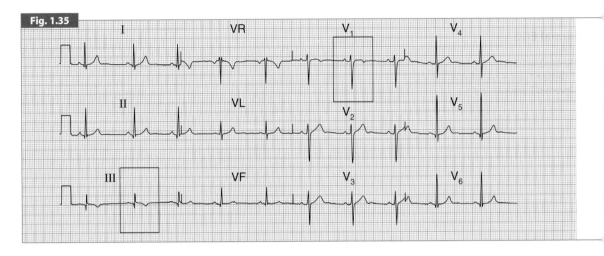

Fig. 1.36

Normal ECG during inspiration

Inspiration

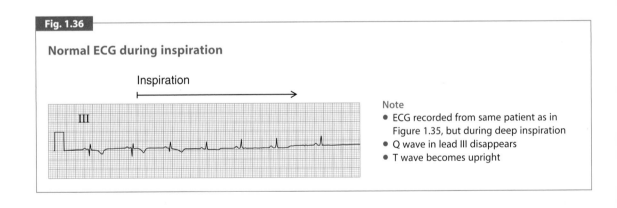

Note
- ECG recorded from same patient as in Figure 1.35, but during deep inspiration
- Q wave in lead III disappears
- T wave becomes upright

Normal ECG

Note
- Small Q wave in lead III but not VF
- Inverted T wave in lead III but upright T wave in VF
- Inverted T wave in lead V_1

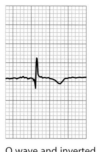

Q wave and inverted
T wave in lead III

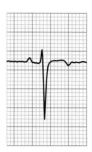

Inverted T wave in
lead V_1

T wave inversion in lead VL as well as in VR can be normal, particularly if the P wave in lead VL is inverted. The ECG in Figure 1.37 was recorded from a completely healthy young woman.

T wave inversion in leads V_2–V_3 as well as in V_1 occurs in pulmonary embolism and in right ventricular hypertrophy (see Chs 5 and 6) but it can be a normal variant. This is particularly true in black people. The ECG in Figure 1.38 was recorded from a healthy young white man, and that shown in Figure 1.39 from a young black professional footballer. The ECG in Figure 1.40 was recorded from a middle-aged black woman with rather nonspecific chest pain, whose coronary arteries and left ventricle were shown to be entirely normal on catheterization.

Box 1.4 summarizes the situations in which T wave inversion is seen.

Box 1.4 Causes of T wave inversion

- Normal in leads VR, V_1–V_2 and V_3, in black people
- Normal in lead III when the T wave in lead VF is upright
- Ventricular extrasystoles and other ventricular rhythms
- Bundle branch block (right or left)
- Myocardial infarction
- Right or left ventricular hypertrophy
- The Wolff–Parkinson–White syndrome

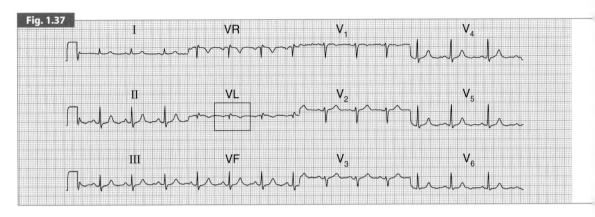

Fig. 1.37

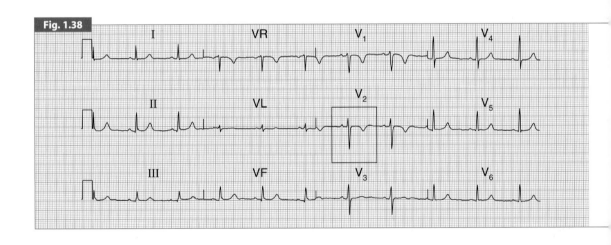

Fig. 1.38

Normal ECG
Note
- Inverted T waves in leads VR, VL
- Inverted P waves in leads VR, VL

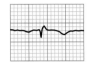

Inverted P and T waves in lead VL

Normal ECG
Note
- T wave inversion in leads VR, V_1–V_2
- Biphasic T wave in lead V_3

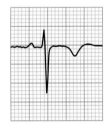

Inverted T wave in lead V_2

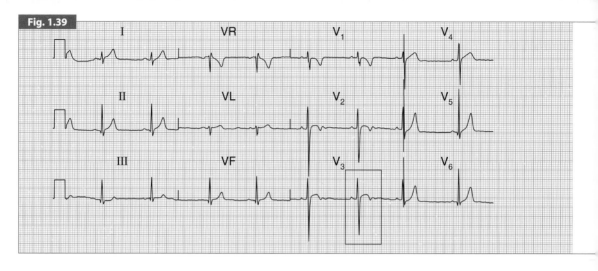

Fig. 1.39

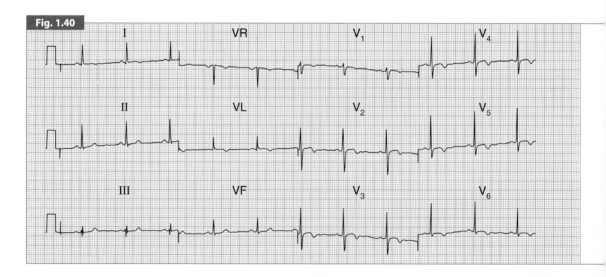

Fig. 1.40

Normal ECG, from a black man
Note
- T wave inversion in leads VR, V_1–V_3
- Early repolarization in leads V_2–V_3

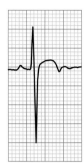

Inverted T wave in lead V_3

Normal ECG, from a black woman
Note
- Sinus rhythm
- T wave inversion in lead VL and all chest leads
- Presumably a normal variant: coronary angiography and echocardiography were normal

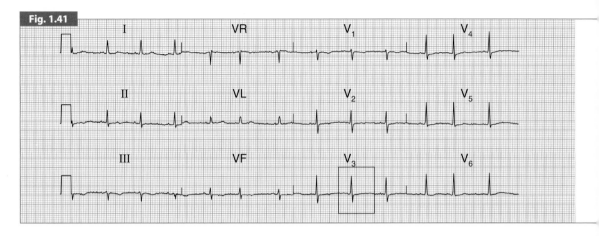

Fig. 1.41

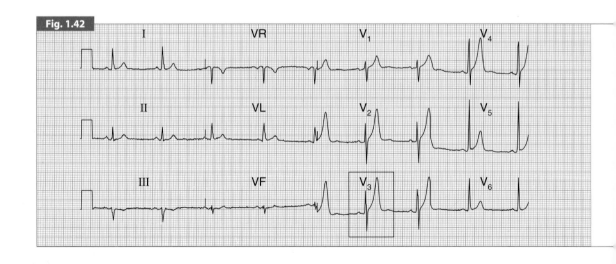

Fig. 1.42

Possibly normal ECG

Note

- Sinus rhythm
- Normal axis
- Normal QRS complexes
- T wave flattening in all chest leads
- T wave inversion in leads III, VF
- In an asymptomatic patient, these changes are not necessarily significant

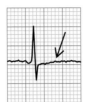

Flattened T wave in lead V₃

Normal ECG

Note

- Sinus rhythm
- Normal axis
- Normal QRS complexes
- Very tall and peaked T wave

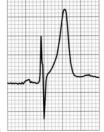

Tall peaked T wave in lead V₃

Generalized flattening of the T waves with a normal QT interval is best described as 'nonspecific'. In a patient without symptoms and whose heart is clinically normal, the finding has little prognostic significance. This was the case with the patient whose ECG is shown in Figure 1.41. In patients with symptoms suggestive of cardiovascular disease, however, such an ECG would require further investigation.

Peaked T waves are one of the features of hyperkalaemia, but they can also be very prominent in healthy people (Fig. 1.42). Tall and peaked T waves are sometimes seen in the early stages of a myocardial infarction, when they are described as 'hyperacute'. They are, however, an extremely unreliable sign of infarction.

The T wave is the most variable part of the ECG. It may become inverted in some leads simply by hyperventilation associated with anxiety.

45

Fig. 1.43

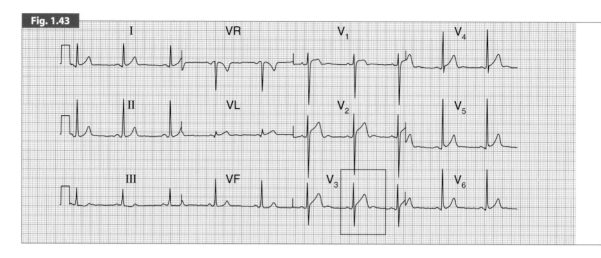

Fig 1.44

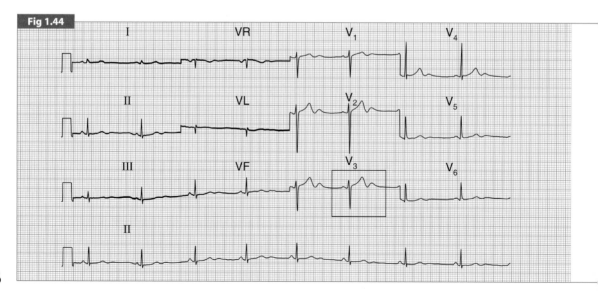

Normal ECG

Note

- Prominent U waves following normal T waves in leads V$_2$–V$_4$

An extra hump on the end of the T wave, a 'U' wave, is characteristic of hypokalaemia. However, U waves are commonly seen in the anterior chest leads of normal ECGs (Fig. 1.43), where they can be remarkably prominent (Fig. 1.44). It is thought that they represent repolarization of the papillary muscles. A U wave is probably only important if it follows a flat T wave.

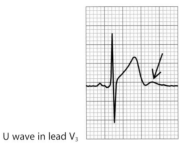

U wave in lead V$_3$

Normal ECG

Note

- Very large U waves following normal T waves in leads V$_1$–V$_4$

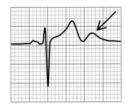

Very large U wave in lead V$_3$

THE QT INTERVAL

The QT interval (from the Q wave to the end of the T wave) varies with the heart rate, gender and time of day. There are several different ways of correcting the QT interval for heart rate, but the simplest is Bazett's formula. In this, the corrected QT interval (QT$_c$) is calculated by:

$$QT_c = \frac{QT}{\sqrt{(R-R \text{ interval})}}$$

An alternative is Fridericia's correction, in which QT$_c$ is the QT interval divided by the cube root of the R–R interval. It is uncertain which of the corrections is clinically more important.

The upper limit of the normal QT$_c$ interval is longer in women than in men, and increases with age. Its precise limit is uncertain, but is usually taken (following Bazett's correction) as 450 ms for adult men and 470 ms for adult women.

THE ECG IN ATHLETES

Any of the normal variations discussed above can be found in athletes. There can be changes in rhythm and/or ECG pattern, and the ECGs of athletes may

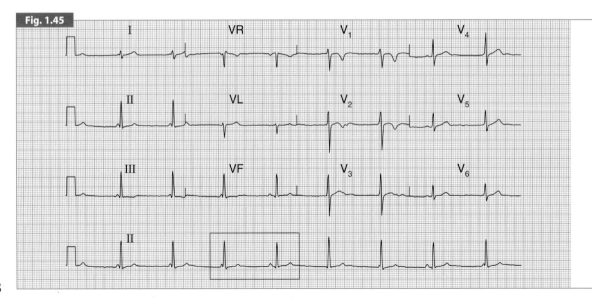

Fig. 1.45

also show some features that might be considered abnormal in non-athletic subjects, but are normal in athletes (see Box 1.5). Figure 1.45 shows the short and varying PR interval of an 'accelerated idionodal rhythm' (also known as a 'wandering atrial pace-maker'). Here the sinus node rate has slowed, and the heart rate is controlled by the AV node, which is discharging faster than the SA node.

The ECGs in Figures 1.45, 1.46 and 1.47 were all recorded during the screening examinations of healthy young footballers.

Box 1.5 Possible ECG features of healthy athletes

Variations in rhythm
- Sinus bradycardia
- Marked sinus arrhythmia
- Junctional rhythm
- 'Wandering' atrial pacemaker
- First degree block
- Wenckebach phenomenon
- Second degree block

Variations in ECG pattern
- Tall P waves
- Prominent septal Q waves
- Tall R waves and deep S waves
- Counterclockwise rotation
- Slight ST segment elevation
- Tall symmetrical T waves
- T wave inversion, especially in lateral leads
- Biphasic T waves
- Prominent U waves

Normal ECG with accelerated idionodal rhythm

Note
- SA node stimulates the atria at a constant rate of 50/min
- Ventricular rate is slightly faster than the atrial rate
- Narrow QRS complexes, originating in the AV node
- QRS complexes appear to 'overtake' the P waves, which are not suppressed – causing an apparent variation in the PR interval

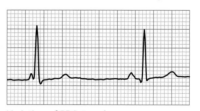

Variation of PR interval

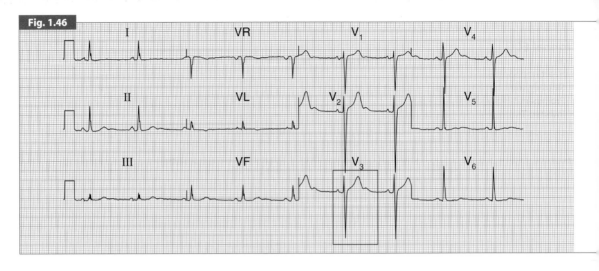

Fig. 1.46

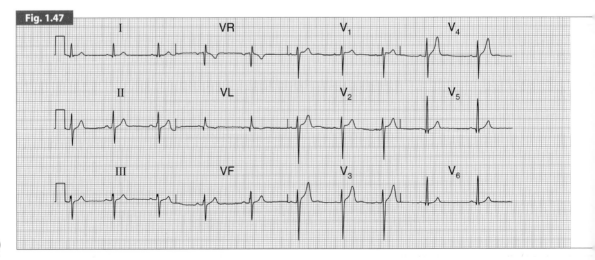

Fig. 1.47

Normal ECG
Note
- Heart rate 53/min
- Sinus rhythm
- Prominent U waves in leads V_2–V_5
- Inverted T waves in lead VL

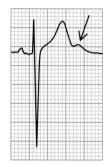

U wave in lead V_3

Normal ECG
Note
- Sinus rhythm
- Left axis deviation
- Septal Q waves in leads V_5–V_6

Fig. 1.48

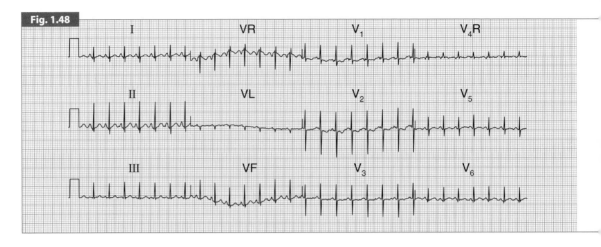

THE ECG IN PREGNANCY

Minor changes in the ECG are commonly seen in pregnancy (see Box 1.6). Ventricular extrasystoles are almost universal.

THE ECG IN CHILDREN

The normal heart rate in the first year of life is 140–160/min, falling slowly to about 80/min by puberty. Sinus arrhythmia is usually quite marked in children.

At birth, the muscle of the right ventricle is as thick as that of the left ventricle. The ECG of a normal child in the first year of life has a pattern that would indicate right ventricular hypertrophy in an adult. The ECG in Figure 1.48 was recorded from a normal 1-month-old child.

Box 1.6 Possible ECG features in pregnancy

- Sinus tachycardia
- Supraventricular and ventricular extrasystoles
- Nonspecific ST segment/T wave changes

The changes suggestive of right ventricular hypertrophy disappear during the first few years of life. All the features other than the inverted T waves in leads V_1 and V_2 should have disappeared by the age of 2 years, and the adult ECG pattern should have developed by the age of 10 years. In general, if the infant ECG pattern persists beyond the age of 2 years, then right ventricular hypertrophy is indeed present. If the normal adult pattern is present in the first year of life, then left ventricular hypertrophy is present.

The ECG changes associated with childhood are summarized in Box 1.7.

Normal ECG, from a child 1 month old

Note

- Heart rate 170/min
- Sinus rhythm
- Normal axis
- Dominant R waves in lead V_1
- Inverted T waves in leads V_1–V_2
- Biphasic T waves in lead V_3
- Lead V_4R (a position on the chest equivalent to V_4, but on the right side) has been recorded instead of V_4

Box 1.7 **The ECG in normal children**

At birth

- Sinus tachycardia
- Right axis deviation
- Dominant R waves in lead V_1
- Deep S waves in lead V_6
- T waves inverted in leads V_1–V_4

At 1 year of age

- Sinus tachycardia
- Right axis deviation
- Dominant R waves in lead V_1
- T waves inverted in leads V_1–V_2

At 2 years of age

- Normal axis
- S waves greater than R waves in lead V_1
- T waves inverted in leads V_1–V_2

At 5 years of age

- Normal QRS complexes
- T waves still inverted in leads V_1–V_2

At 10 years of age

- Adult pattern

FREQUENCY OF ECG ABNORMALITIES IN HEALTHY PEOPLE

The ECG findings we have discussed so far can all be considered to be within the normal range. Certain findings are undoubtedly abnormal as far as the ECG is concerned, yet do occur in apparently healthy people.

The frequency with which abnormalities are detected depends on the population studied: most abnormalities are found least often in healthy young people recruited to the armed services, and become progressively more common in populations of increasing age. An exception to this rule is that frequent ventricular extrasystoles are very common in pregnancy. The frequency of right and left bundle branch block has been found to be 0.3% and 0.1% respectively in populations of young recruits to the services, but in older working populations these abnormalities have been detected in 2% and 0.7% respectively of apparently healthy people.

WHAT TO DO ▶

When an apparently healthy subject has an ECG record that appears abnormal, the most important thing is not to cause unnecessary alarm. There are four questions to ask:

1. Does the ECG really come from that individual? If so, is he or she really asymptomatic and are the findings of the physical examination really normal?
2. Is the ECG really abnormal or is it within the normal range?
3. If the ECG is indeed abnormal, what are the implications for the patient?
4. What further investigations are needed?

THE RANGE OF NORMALITY

Normal variations in the P waves, QRS complexes and T waves have been described in detail. T wave changes usually give the most trouble in terms of ECG interpretation, because changes in repolarization occur in many different circumstances, and in any individual, and variations in T wave morphology can occur from day to day.

Box 1.8 lists some of the ECG patterns that can be accepted as normal in healthy patients, and some that must be regarded with suspicion.

THE PROGNOSIS OF PATIENTS WITH AN ABNORMAL ECG

In general, the prognosis is related to the patient's clinical history and to the findings on physical examination, rather than to the ECG. An abnormal ECG is much more significant in a patient with symptoms and signs of heart disease than it is in a truly healthy subject. In the absence of any other evidence of heart disease, the prognosis of an individual with one of the more common ECG abnormalities is as follows.

CONDUCTION DEFECTS

First degree block (especially when the PR interval is only slightly prolonged) has little effect on prognosis. Second and third degree block indicate heart disease and the prognosis is worse, though the congenital form of complete block is less serious than the acquired form in adults.

Left anterior hemiblock has a good prognosis, as does right bundle branch block (RBBB). The presence of left bundle branch block (LBBB) in the absence of other manifestations of cardiac disease is associated

Box 1.8 **Variations in the normal ECG in adults**

Rhythm
- Marked sinus arrhythmia, with escape beats
- Lack of sinus arrhythmia (normal with increasing age)
- Supraventricular extrasystoles
- Ventricular extrasystoles

P wave
- Normally inverted in lead VR
- May be inverted in lead VL

Cardiac axis
- Minor right axis deviation in tall people

QRS complexes in the chest leads
- Slight dominance of R wave in lead V_1, provided there is no other evidence of right ventricular hypertrophy or posterior infarction
- The R wave in the lateral chest leads may exceed 25 mm in thin fit young people
- Partial right bundle branch block (RSR[1] pattern, with QRS complexes less than 120 ms)
- Septal Q waves in leads III, VL, V_5–V_6

ST segment
- Raised in anterior leads following an S wave (high take-off ST segment)
- Depressed in pregnancy
- Nonspecific upward-sloping depression

T wave
- Inverted in lead VR and often in V_1
- Inverted in leads V_2–V_3, or even V_4 in black people
- May invert with hyperventilation
- Peaked, especially if the T waves are tall

U wave
- Normal in anterior leads when the T wave is not flattened

with about a 30% increase in the risk of death compared with that of individuals with a normal ECG. The risk of death doubles if a subject known to have a normal ECG suddenly develops LBBB, even if there are no symptoms – the ECG change presumably indicates progressive cardiac disease, probably most often ischaemia. Bifascicular block seldom progresses to complete block, but is always an indication of underlying heart disease – the prognosis is therefore relatively poor compared to that of patients with LBBB alone.

ARRHYTHMIAS

Supraventricular extrasystoles are of no importance whatsoever. Ventricular extrasystoles are almost universal, but when frequent or multiform they indicate populations with a statistically increased risk of death, presumably because in some people they indicate subclinical heart disease. The increased risk to an individual is, however, insignificant and there is no evidence that treating ventricular extrasystoles prolongs survival.

Atrial fibrillation is frequently the result of rheumatic or ischaemic heart disease or cardiomyopathy, and the prognosis is then relatively poor. In about one third of individuals with atrial fibrillation no cardiac disease can be demonstrated. However, even in these people the risk of death is increased by three or four times, and the risk of stroke is increased perhaps tenfold, compared with people of the same age whose hearts are in sinus rhythm.

FURTHER INVESTIGATIONS

Complex and expensive investigations are seldom justified in asymptomatic patients whose hearts are clinically normal, but who have been found to have an abnormal ECG.

An echocardiogram should be recorded in all patients with bundle branch block, to assess the size and function of the individual heart chambers. Patients with LBBB may have a dilated cardiomyopathy, and the echocardiogram will then show a dilated left ventricle which contracts poorly. Alternatively they may have ischaemia, and the echocardiogram will show some segments of the left ventricle failing to contract or contracting poorly. Patients with LBBB may also have unsuspected aortic stenosis. Patients with RBBB may have an atrial septal defect or pulmonary hypertension, but quite frequently the echocardiogram shows no abnormality.

Echocardiography may be helpful in establishing the cause of T wave inversion, which might be due to ischaemia, ventricular hypertrophy or cardiomyopathy.

Patients with frequent ventricular extrasystoles seldom need detailed investigation, but if there is any question of underlying heart disease an echocardiogram may help to exclude the possibility of a cardiomyopathy. It is also worth checking their blood haemoglobin level.

In patients with atrial fibrillation, an echocardiogram is useful for defining or excluding structural abnormalities, and for studying left ventricular function. An echocardiogram is indicated if there is anything that might suggest rheumatic heart disease. Since atrial fibrillation can be the only manifestation of thyrotoxicosis, thyroid function must be checked. Atrial fibrillation may also be the result of alcoholism, and this may be denied by the patient, so it may be fair to check liver function.

Table 1.1 shows investigations that should be considered in the case of various cardiac rhythms and indicates which underlying diseases may be present.

TREATMENT OF ASYMPTOMATIC ECG ABNORMALITIES

It is always the patient who should be treated, not the ECG. The prognosis of patients with complete heart block is improved by permanent pacing, but that of patients with other degrees of block is not. Ventricular extrasystoles should not be treated because of the risk of the pro-arrhythmic effects of antiarrhythmic drugs. Atrial fibrillation need not be treated if the ventricular rate is reasonable, but anticoagulation must be considered in all cases. In the case of patients with valve disease and atrial fibrillation, however, anticoagulant treatment is essential.

Table 1.1 Investigations in apparently healthy people with an abnormal ECG

ECG appearance	Diagnosis to be excluded	Possible investigations
Sinus tachycardia	Thyrotoxicosis Anaemia Changes in heart size ⎫ Heart failure ⎬ Systolic dysfunction ⎭	Thyroid function Haemoglobin Echocardiogram
Sinus bradycardia	Myxoedema	Thyroid function
Frequent ventricular extrasystoles	Left ventricular dysfunction Anaemia	Echocardiogram Haemoglobin
Right bundle branch block	Heart size Lung disease Atrial septal defect	Echocardiogram
Left bundle branch block	Heart size Aortic stenosis Cardiomyopathy Ischaemia	Echocardiogram
T wave abnormalities	High or low potassium or calcium Ventricular systolic dysfunction ⎫ Hypertrophic cardiomyopathy ⎬ Ischaemia	Electrolytes Echocardiogram Exercise test Myocardial perfusion scan
Atrial fibrillation	Thyrotoxicosis Alcoholism Valve disease, ventricular ⎫ and left atrial dimensions ⎬ Myxoma ⎭	Thyroid function Liver function Echocardiogram

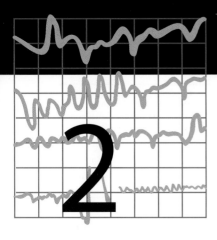

2

The ECG in patients with palpitations and syncope: between attacks

The clinical history and physical examination   **59**

Palpitations   59

Dizziness and syncope   60

Physical examination   64

The ECG   **64**

Syncope due to cardiac disease other than arrhythmias   64

Patients with possible tachycardias   69

Patients with possible bradycardias   82

Ambulatory ECG recording   96

The ECG is of paramount importance for the diagnosis of arrhythmias. Many arrhythmias are not noticed by the patient, but often they cause symptoms. These symptoms are often transient, and the patient may be completely well at the time he or she consults a doctor. Obtaining an ECG during a symptomatic episode is then the only certain way of making a diagnosis, but as always the history and physical examination are also extremely important. The main purpose of the history and examination is to help decide whether a patient's symptoms could be the result of an arrhythmia, and whether the patient has a cardiac or other disease that may cause an arrhythmia.

THE CLINICAL HISTORY AND PHYSICAL EXAMINATION

PALPITATIONS

'Palpitations' mean different things to different patients, but a general definition would be 'an awareness of the heartbeat'. Arrhythmias, fast or slow, can cause poor organ perfusion and so lead to syncope (a word used to describe all sorts of collapse), breathlessness and angina. Some rhythms can be identified from a patient's description, such as:

- A patient recognizes sinus tachycardia because it feels like the palpitations that he or she associates with anxiety or exercise.

- Extrasystoles are described as the heart 'jumping' or 'missing a beat'. It is not possible to distinguish between supraventricular and ventricular extrasystoles from a patient's description, although they can be differentiated from an ECG.

- A paroxysmal tachycardia begins suddenly and sometimes stops suddenly. The heart rate is often 'too fast to count'. Severe attacks are associated with dizziness, breathlessness and chest pain.

Table 2.1 compares the symptoms associated with sinus tachycardia and a paroxysmal tachycardia, and shows how a diagnosis can be made from the history. Note that a heart rate between 140/min and 160/min may be associated with either sinus or paroxysmal tachycardia.

Table 2.1 Diagnosis of sinus tachycardia or paroxysmal tachycardia from a patient's symptoms

Symptoms	Sinus tachycardia	Paroxysmal tachycardia
Timing of initial attack	Attacks probably began recently	Attacks probably began in teens or early adult life
Associations of attack	Exercise, anxiety	Usually no associations, but occasionally exercise-induced
Rate of start of palpitations	Slow build-up	Sudden onset
Rate of end of palpitations	'Die away'	Classically sudden, but often 'die away'
Heart rate	<140/min	>160/min
Associated symptoms	Paraesthesia due to hyperventilation	Chest pain Breathlessness Dizziness Syncope
Ways of terminating attacks	Relaxation	Breath holding Valsalva's manoeuvre

DIZZINESS AND SYNCOPE

These symptoms may have a cardiovascular or a neurological cause. Remember that cerebral hypoxia, however caused, may lead to a seizure, and that can make the differentiation between cardiac and neurological syncope very difficult. Syncope is defined as 'a transient loss of consciousness characterized by unresponsiveness and loss of postural tone, with spontaneous recovery and not requiring specific resuscitative intervention'.

Figure 2.1 shows an EEG that was being recorded in a 46-year-old woman with episodes of limb shaking, suspected of being generalized tonic–clonic seizures. She lost awareness during events, and had violent limb shaking for several seconds as she came round. She felt nauseated, but was rapidly reorientated. By chance, she had one of her 'attacks' while her EEG was being recorded, and from the ECG being routinely recorded in parallel, it became clear that the problem was not seizures, but periods of asystole – in this case lasting about 15 s. The numbered arrows in Figure 2.1 mark significant features. The recording begins with a routine period of hyperventilation, with the EEG showing an eye blink in the anterior leads and the ECG showing sinus rhythm. There are then (at arrow 1 on the record) one (or possibly two) ventricular extrasystoles, followed by a narrow complex beat (probably sinus) and another ventricular extrasystole, with a different configuration from the previous ones. Asystole follows, and after 7–8 s (at arrow 2) there is global EEG slowing, and the patient became unresponsive. After 4 s (at arrow 3), there is global attenuation (reduction in signals) in the EEG and after another 3 s, there is an escape beat whose morphology suggests a ventricular origin. This is followed by a beat with a narrow QRS complex and possibly an inverted T wave, and then there is gross artefact due to the ECG lead being checked. During that period, sinus rhythm was restored. There was then (at arrow 4) global EEG slowing for 5 s, followed by (at arrow 5) violent limb thrashing for about 12 s as the patient regained consciousness – these movements were not clonic, and were thought to represent anxiety or fear. Normal EEG and ECG activity were then resumed (at arrow 6).

Some causes of syncope are summarized in Box 2.1.

Table 2.2 shows some clinical features of syncope, and possible causes.

Box 2.1 Cardiovascular causes of syncope

Obstructed blood flow in heart or lungs
- Aortic stenosis
- Pulmonary embolus
- Pulmonary hypertension
- Hypertrophic cardiomyopathy
- Pericardial tamponade
- Atrial myxoma

Arrhythmias
- Tachycardias: patient is usually aware of a fast heartbeat before becoming dizzy
- Bradycardias: slow heart rates are often not appreciated. A classical cause of syncope is a Stokes–Adams attack, due to a very slow ventricular rate in patients with complete heart block. A Stokes–Adams attack can be recognized because the patient is initially pale but flushes red on recovery

Postural hypotension, occurring immediately on standing
Seen with:
- Loss of blood volume
- Autonomic nervous system disease (e.g. diabetes, Shy–Drager syndrome, amyloid neuropathy)
- Patients being treated with antihypertensive drugs

Neurally-mediated reflex syncopal syndromes
- Vasovagal (neurocardiogenic) (simple faints)
- Situational (e.g. after coughing, sneezing, gastrointestinal stimulation of various sorts, post-micturition)
- Carotid sinus hypersensitivity

Table 2.2 Diagnosis of causes of syncope

Symptoms and signs	Possible diagnosis
Family history of sudden death	Long QT syndrome, Brugada syndrome, hypertrophic cardiomyopathy
Caused by unpleasant stimuli, prolonged standing, hot places (situational syncope)	Vasovagal syncope
Occurs within seconds or minutes of standing	Orthostatic hypotension
Temporal relation to medication	Orthostatic hypotension
Occurs during exertion	Obstruction to blood flow (e.g. aortic stenosis, pulmonary hypertension)
Occurs with head rotation or pressure on neck	Carotid sinus hypersensitivity
Confusion for more than 5 min afterwards	Seizure
Tonic–clonic movements, automatism	Seizure
Frequent attacks, usually unobserved, with somatic symptoms	Psychiatric illness
Symptoms or signs suggesting cardiac disease	Cardiac disease

Fig. 2.1

EEG recorded during a syncopal attack

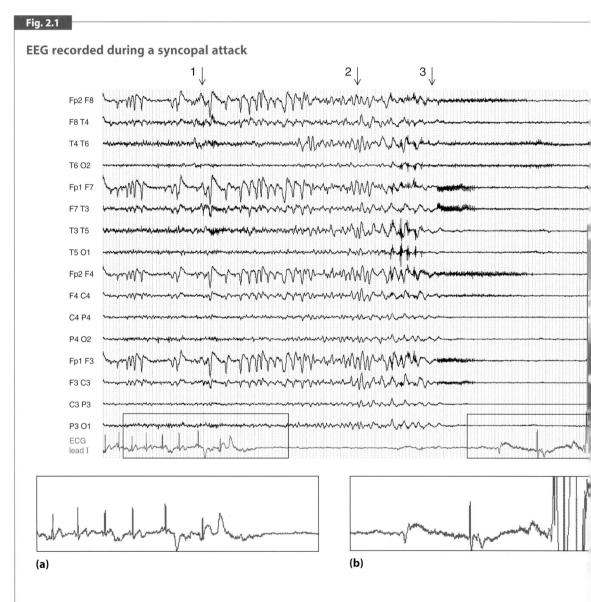

(a)
(b)

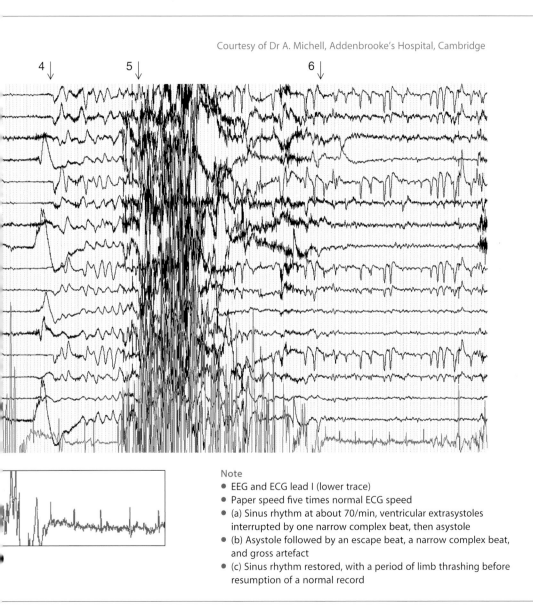

Note

- EEG and ECG lead I (lower trace)
- Paper speed five times normal ECG speed
- (a) Sinus rhythm at about 70/min, ventricular extrasystoles interrupted by one narrow complex beat, then asystole
- (b) Asystole followed by an escape beat, a narrow complex beat, and gross artefact
- (c) Sinus rhythm restored, with a period of limb thrashing before resumption of a normal record

PHYSICAL EXAMINATION

If the patient has no symptoms at the time of the examination, look for:

- Evidence of any heart disease that might cause an arrhythmia
- Evidence of non-cardiac disease that might cause an arrhythmia
- Evidence of cardiovascular disease that might cause syncope without an arrhythmia
- Evidence (from the history or examination) of neurological disease.

It is only possible to make a confident diagnosis that an arrhythmia is the cause of palpitations or syncope if an ECG recording of the arrhythmia can be obtained at the time of the patient's symptoms. If the patient is asymptomatic at the time of examination, it may be worth arranging for an ECG to be recorded during an attack of palpitations, or to be recorded continuously, in the hope that an episode of the arrhythmia will be detected.

THE ECG

Even when the patient is asymptomatic, the resting ECG can be very helpful, as summarized in Table 2.3.

SYNCOPE DUE TO CARDIAC DISEASE OTHER THAN ARRHYTHMIAS

The ECG may indicate that syncopal attacks have a cardiovascular cause other than an arrhythmia.

ECG evidence of left ventricular hypertrophy or of left bundle branch block may suggest that syncope is due to aortic stenosis. The ECGs in Figures 2.2 and 2.3 were recorded from patients who had syncopal attacks on exercise due to severe aortic stenosis.

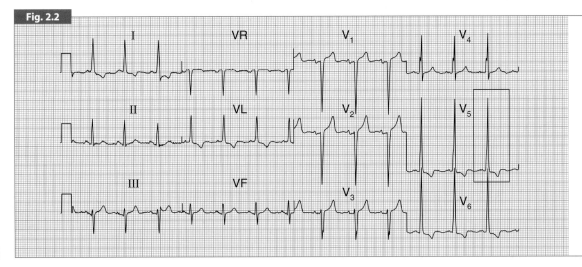

Fig. 2.2

Table 2.3 ECG features between attacks of palpitations or syncope

ECG appearance	Possible cause of symptoms
ECG completely normal	Symptoms may not be due to a primary arrhythmia – consider anxiety, epilepsy, atrial myxoma or carotid sinus hypersensitivity
ECGs that suggest cardiac disease	Left ventricular hypertrophy or left bundle branch block – aortic stenosis Right ventricular hypertrophy – pulmonary hypertension Anterior T wave inversion – hypertrophic cardiomyopathy
ECGs that suggest intermittent tachyarrhythmia	Left atrial hypertrophy – mitral stenosis, so possibly atrial fibrillation Pre-excitation syndromes Long QT syndrome Flat T waves suggest hypokalaemia Digoxin effect – ?digoxin toxicity
ECGs that suggest intermittent bradyarrhythmia	Second degree block First degree block plus bundle branch block Digoxin effect

Left ventricular hypertrophy
Note
- Sinus rhythm
- Bifid P waves suggest left atrial hypertrophy (best seen in leads V_4–V_5)
- Normal axis
- Tall R waves and deep S waves
- T waves inverted in leads I, VL, V_5–V_6

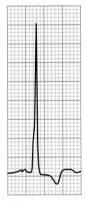

Tall R wave, inverted T wave in lead V_5

Fig. 2.3

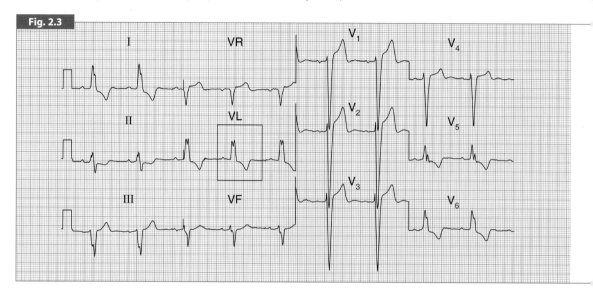

Fig. 2.4

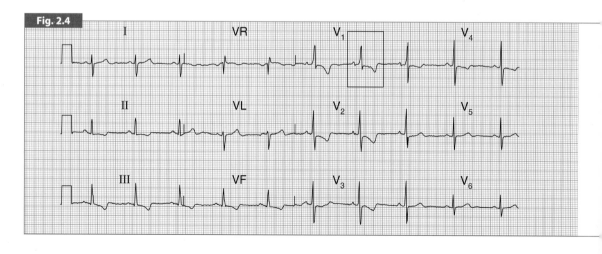

Left bundle branch block

Note
- Sinus rhythm
- Slight PR interval prolongation (212 ms)
- Broad QRS complexes
- 'M' pattern in lateral leads
- T wave inversion in leads I, VL, V$_5$–V$_6$

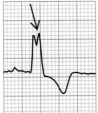

M pattern of left bundle branch block in lead VL

ECG evidence of right ventricular hypertrophy suggests thromboembolic pulmonary hypertension. The ECG in Figure 2.4 is that of a middle-aged woman with dizziness on exertion, due to multiple pulmonary emboli.

Syncope due to hypertrophic cardiomyopathy (Fig. 2.5) may be associated with a characteristic ECG (Fig. 2.6) that resembles that of patients with an anterior non-ST segment elevation myocardial infarction (NSTEMI) (compare with Fig. 5.23, p. 240). With hypertrophic cardiomyopathy, the T wave inversion is usually more pronounced than with an NSTEMI, but differentiation really depends on the clinical picture, not on the ECG appearance. Hypertrophic cardiomyopathy can cause syncope due to obstruction to outflow from the left ventricle, or can cause symptomatic arrhythmias.

Right ventricular hypertrophy

Note
- Sinus rhythm
- Right axis deviation
- Dominant R waves in lead V$_1$
- Inverted T waves in leads V$_1$–V$_4$

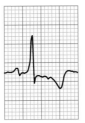

Dominant R wave in lead V$_1$

Fig 2.5

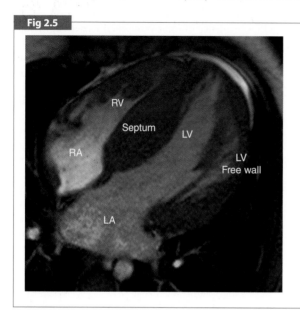

MR image of a heart with hypertrophic cardiomyopathy
Note
- RA – right atrium
- RV – right ventricular cavity
- Septum – interventricular septum
- LV – left ventricular cavity
- LA – left atrium
- LV free wall – left ventricular myocardium

Fig. 2.6

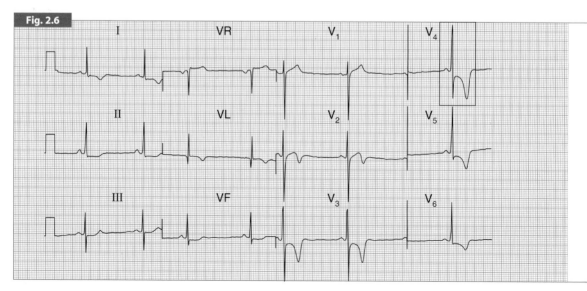

PATIENTS WITH POSSIBLE TACHYCARDIAS

MITRAL STENOSIS

Mitral stenosis leads to atrial fibrillation, but when the heart is still in sinus rhythm the presence of the characteristics of left atrial hypertrophy on the ECG may give a clue that paroxysmal atrial fibrillation is occurring (Fig. 2.7).

PRE-EXCITATION SYNDROMES

Normal conduction between the atria and ventricles involves the uniform spread of the depolarization wave front in a constant direction, down the bundle of His. In the pre-excitation syndromes, an abnormal additional pathway, or multiple pathways, connect the atria and ventricles. These accessory pathways bypass the AV node, where normal conduction is delayed, and

therefore conduct more rapidly than the normal pathway. The anatomical combination of the normal AV node–His bundle pathway and the accessory pathway creates a potential circuit around which excitation may spread, causing a 're-entry' tachycardia (Ch. 3, p. 105).

The Wolff–Parkinson–White syndrome

In the Wolff–Parkinson–White (WPW) syndrome, an accessory pathway (the 'bundle of Kent') connects either the left atrium and left ventricle, or the right atrium and right ventricle. Conduction may at times occur only through the normal His bundle pathway, so the QRS complexes will be normal and narrow; the accessory pathway is then said to be concealed. At other times, conduction may occur through both pathways simultaneously, but the heart will remain in sinus rhythm if conduction occurs in a forward direction via both the AV node–His bundle pathway and the accessory pathway. The faster conduction down the accessory pathway causes part of the ventricle to depolarize early, resulting in a short PR interval and a slurred upstroke to the QRS complex (delta wave), causing a wide QRS complex.

With a left-sided accessory pathway, the ECG shows a dominant R wave in lead V_1. This is called the 'type A' pattern (Fig. 2.8). This pattern can easily be mistaken for right ventricular hypertrophy, the differentiation being made by the presence or absence of a short PR interval.

Hypertrophic cardiomyopathy

Note
- Sinus rhythm
- Marked T wave inversion in leads V_3–V_6

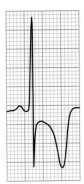

Inverted T wave in lead V_4

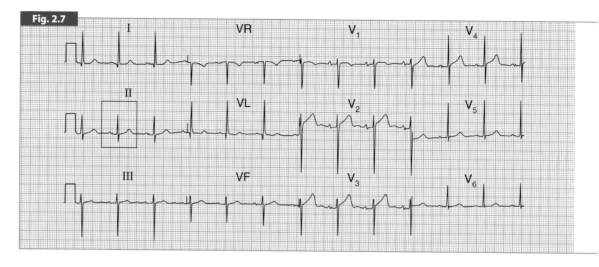

Fig. 2.7

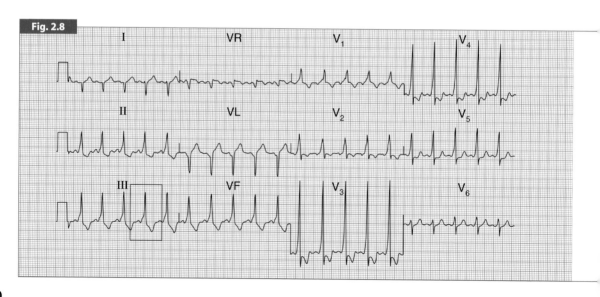

Fig. 2.8

Left atrial hypertrophy

Note

- Sinus rhythm
- Bifid P waves, most clearly seen in leads I, II, V_3–V_5

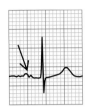

Bifid P wave in lead II

The Wolff–Parkinson–White syndrome, type A

Note

- Sinus rhythm
- Short PR interval
- Broad QRS complexes
- Dominant R wave in lead V_1
- Slurred upstroke to QRS complexes – the delta wave
- Inverted T waves in leads II, III, VF, V_1–V_4

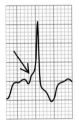

Delta wave in lead III

Fig. 2.9

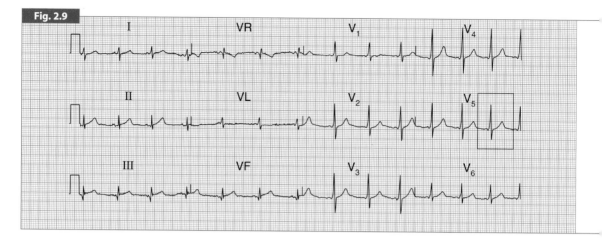

The ECG in Figure 2.9 is from a young man who complained of symptoms that sounded like paroxysmal tachycardia. His ECG shows the WPW syndrome type A, but it would be quite easy to miss the short PR interval unless the whole of the 12-lead trace were carefully inspected. The short PR interval and delta waves are most obvious in leads V_4 and V_5.

When the accessory pathway is on the right side of the heart, there is no dominant R wave in lead V_1, and this is called the 'type B' pattern (Fig. 2.10).

ECGs indicating pre-excitation of the WPW type are found in approximately 1 in every 3000 healthy young people. Only half of these ever have an episode of tachycardia, and many have only very occasional attacks.

The ECG features associated with the WPW syndrome are summarized in Box 2.2.

The Lown–Ganong–Levine syndrome

Where an accessory pathway connects the atria to the bundle of His rather than to the right or left ventricle, there will be a short PR interval but the QRS complex will be normal. This is called the Lown–Ganong–Levine (LGL) syndrome (Fig. 2.11). This syndrome must be differentiated from accelerated idionodal rhythm, where the PR interval varies (see p. 49 and Fig. 1.45).

The Wolff–Parkinson–White syndrome, type A

Note

- Sinus rhythm
- Short PR interval, especially obvious in leads V_3–V_5
- Slurred upstroke to QRS complexes, obvious in leads V_3–V_5 but not obvious in the limb leads
- Dominant R wave in lead V_1
- No T wave inversion in the anterior leads (cf. Fig. 2.8)

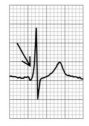

Delta wave in lead V_5

Box 2.2 The Wolff–Parkinson–White syndrome: ECG features

- Short PR interval
- Wide QRS complexes with delta wave with normal terminal segment
- ST segment/T wave changes
- Left-sided pathway (type A): dominant R waves in leads V_1–V_6
- Right-sided pathway (type B): dominant S wave in lead V_1, and sometimes, anterior T wave inversion
- Arrhythmias (narrow or wide complex)
- Arrhythmia with wide, irregular complex suggests the WPW syndrome with atrial fibrillation

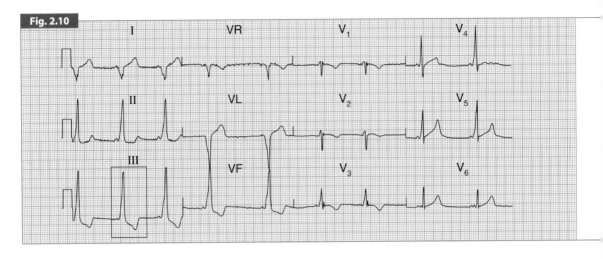

Fig. 2.10

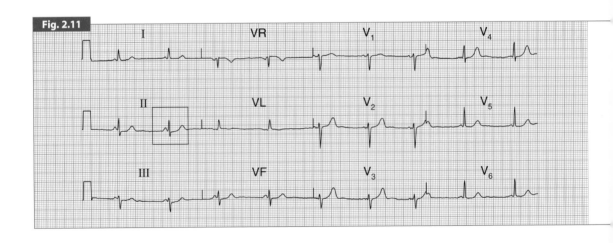

Fig. 2.11

The Wolff–Parkinson–White syndrome, type B

Note
- Sinus rhythm
- Short PR interval
- Broad QRS complexes with delta waves
- No dominant R waves in lead V_1 (cf. Figs 2.8 and 2.9)
- T wave inversion in leads III, VF, V_3

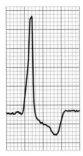

Short PR interval; broad QRS complex in lead III

The Lown–Ganong–Levine syndrome

Note
- Sinus rhythm
- Short PR interval
- Normal QRS complexes and P waves

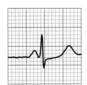

Short PR interval in lead II

75

THE LONG QT SYNDROME

Delayed repolarization occurs for a variety of reasons (Box 2.3), and causes a long QT interval. A prolonged QT interval is associated with paroxysmal ventricular tachycardia, and therefore can be the cause of episodes of collapse or even sudden death. The ventricular tachycardia associated with a prolonged QT interval usually involves a continual change from upright to downward QRS complexes. This is called 'torsade de pointes' (Fig. 2.12), and it usually occurs at times of increased sympathetic nervous system activity.

Several genetic abnormalities have been described that lead to familial prolongation of the QT interval. The ECG in Figure 2.13 is from a 10-year-old girl who suffered from 'fainting' attacks. Her sister had died suddenly; three other siblings and both parents had normal ECGs.

Fig. 2.12

Torsade de pointes ventricular tachycardia

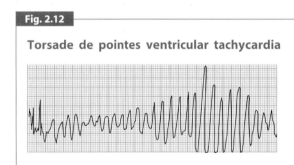

Note
- Broad complex tachycardia at 300/min
- Continually changing shape of QRS complexes

Fig. 2.13

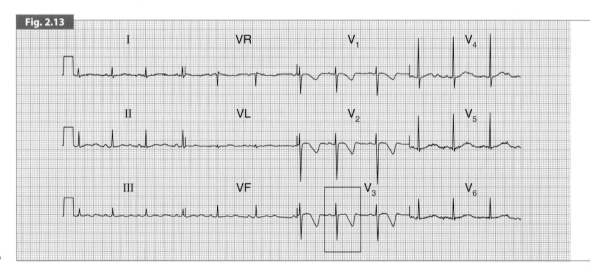

Box 2.3 **Possible causes of a prolonged QT interval**

Congenital
- Jervell–Lange–Nielson syndrome
- Romano–Ward syndrome

Antiarrhythmic drugs
- Quinidine (of historical interest only)
- Procainamide
- Disopyramide
- Amiodarone
- Sotalol

Other drugs
- Tricyclic antidepressants
- Erythromycin

Plasma electrolyte abnormality
- Low potassium
- Low magnesium
- Low calcium

The most common cause of QT prolongation is drug therapy. The ECG in Figure 2.14 is from a patient who had a posterior myocardial infarction (see Ch. 5). He was treated with amiodarone because of recurrent ventricular tachycardias, and developed a prolonged QT interval. Figure 2.15 shows his record 4 months later: the prolonged QT interval reverted to normal when the amiodarone treatment was stopped.

Episodes of symptomatic ventricular tachycardia occur in about 8% of affected subjects each year, and the annual death rate due to arrhythmias is about 1% of patients with a long QT syndrome. The precise relationship between QT_c interval prolongation and the risk of sudden death is unknown; neither is it clear whether prolongation of the QT or QT_c interval is more significant. There is no absolute threshold of risk. However, torsade de pointes ventricular tachycardia seems rare when the QT or QT_c interval is less than 500 ms.

Congenital long QT syndrome
Note
- Sinus rhythm
- Normal axis
- QT interval 520 ms
- Marked T wave inversion in leads V_2–V_4

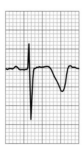

Long QT interval and inverted T wave in lead V_3

Fig. 2.14

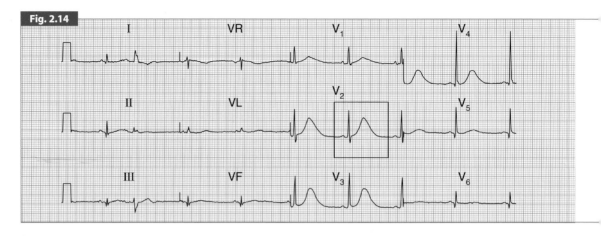

Fig. 2.15

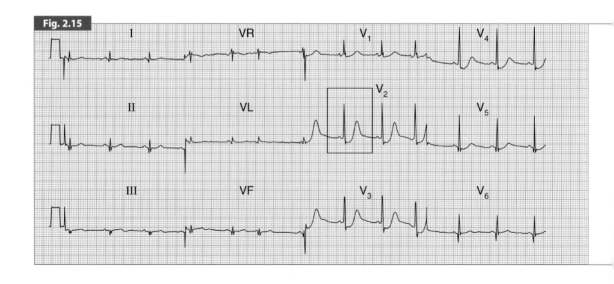

Prolonged QT interval due to amiodarone

Note
- Sinus rhythm
- Normal axis
- Dominant R waves in lead V_1 due to posterior infarction
- QT interval 800 ms
- Bizarre T wave shape in anterior leads

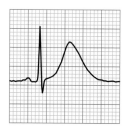

Long QT interval and bizarre T wave in lead V_2

Posterior infarct with normal QT interval

Note
- Same patient as in Figure 2.14
- Sinus rhythm
- Normal axis
- Dominant R waves in lead V_1
- Ischaemic ST segment depression
- Normal QT interval

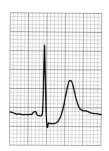

ST segment depression in lead V_2

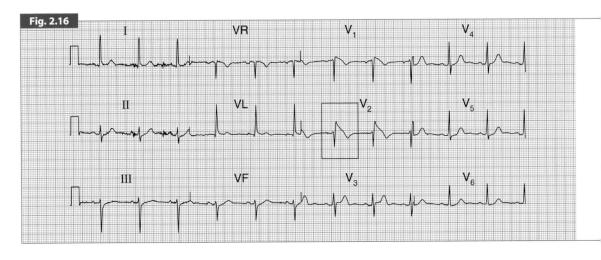

Fig. 2.16

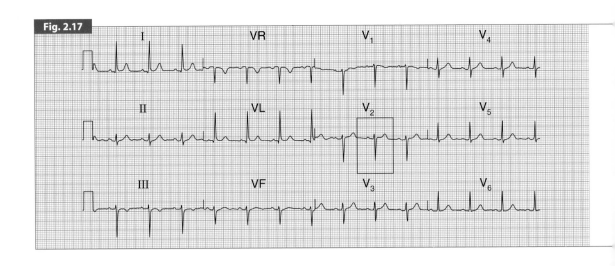

Fig. 2.17

Brugada syndrome
Note
- Sinus rhythm
- Normal axis
- Normal QRS complex duration
- RSR^1 pattern in leads V_1–V_2
- No wide S wave in lead V_6
- Raised, downward-sloping ST segment in leads V_1–V_2

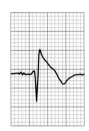

RSR^1 pattern and raised ST segment in lead V_2

Brugada syndrome
Note
- Same patient as in Figure 2.16
- Normal ECG

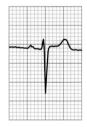

Normal appearance in lead V_2

THE BRUGADA SYNDROME

Sudden collapse due to ventricular tachycardia and fibrillation occurs in a congenital disorder of sodium ion transport called the Brugada syndrome. Between attacks, the ECG superficially resembles that associated with right bundle branch block (RBBB), with an RSR^1 pattern in leads V_1 and V_2 (Fig. 2.16). However, the ST segment in these leads is raised, and there is no wide S wave in lead V_6 as there is in RBBB. The changes are seen in the right ventricular leads because the abnormal sodium channels are predominantly found in the right ventricle. The ECG abnormality can be transient – the ECG in Figure 2.17 was taken a day later from the same patient as in Figure 2.16.

PATIENTS WITH POSSIBLE BRADYCARDIAS

When a patient is asymptomatic, an intermittent brady-cardia can be suspected if the ECG shows any evidence of an escape rhythm or a conduction defect. However, it must be remembered that conduction defects and escape rhythms are quite common in healthy people, and their presence may be coincidental.

ESCAPE RHYTHMS

Myocardial cells are only depolarized when they are stimulated, but the cells of the SA node, those around the AV node (the 'junctional' cells) and those of the conducting pathways all possess the property of spontaneous depolarization or 'automaticity'.

The automaticity of any part of the heart is suppressed by the arrival of a depolarization wave, and so the heart rate is controlled by the region with the highest automatic depolarization frequency. Normally the SA node controls the heart rate because it has thehighest frequency of discharge, but if for any reason this fails, the region with the next highest intrinsic depolarization frequency will emerge as the pacemaker and set up an 'escape' rhythm. The atria and the junctional region have automatic

---

Fig. 2.18

Junctional escape beat

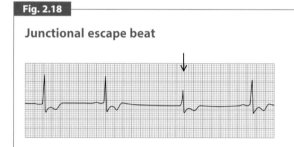

Note
- After two sinus beats there is no P wave
- After an interval there is a narrow QRS complex, with the same configuration as that of the sinus beats but without a preceding P wave
- This is a junctional beat (arrowed)
- Sinus rhythm then reappears

Fig. 2.19

Junctional (escape) rhythm

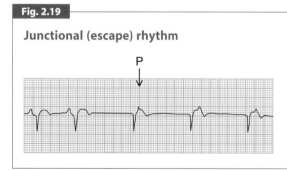

Note
- Two sinus beats are followed by an interval with no P waves
- A junctional rhythm then emerges (with QRS complexes the same as in sinus rhythm)
- A P wave (arrowed) can be seen as a hump on the T wave of the junctional beats: the atria have been depolarized retrogradely

depolarization frequencies of about 50/min, compared with the normal SA node frequency of 60–70/min. If both the SA node and the junctional region fail to depolarize, or if conduction to the ventricles fails, a ventricular focus may emerge, with a rate of 30–40/min; this is classically seen in complete heart block.

Escape beats may be single or may form sustained rhythms. They have the same ECG appearance as the corresponding extrasystoles, but appear late rather than early (Fig. 2.18).

In sustained junctional escape rhythms, atrial activation may be seen as a P wave following the QRS complex (Fig. 2.19). This occurs if depolarization spreads in the opposite direction from normal, from the AV node to the atria, and is called 'retrograde' conduction. Figure 2.20 also shows a junctional escape rhythm.

Figure 2.21 shows a ventricular escape beat.

Fig. 2.20

Junctional (escape) rhythm

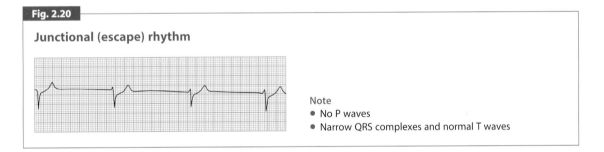

Note
- No P waves
- Narrow QRS complexes and normal T waves

Fig. 2.21

Ventricular escape beat

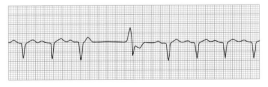

Note
- Three sinus beats are followed by a pause
- There is then a single ventricular beat with a wide QRS complex and an inverted T wave
- Sinus rhythm is then restored

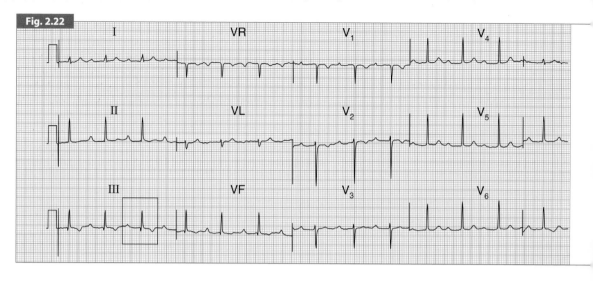

Fig. 2.22

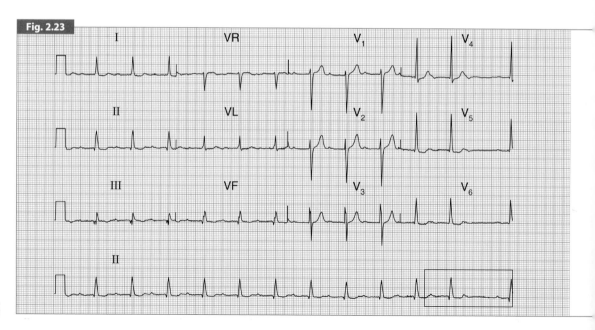

Fig. 2.23

First degree block

Note
- Sinus rhythm
- PR interval 380 ms
- T wave inversion in leads III and VF suggests ischaemia

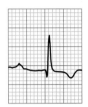

Long PR interval in lead III

SYNCOPE

In a patient with syncopal attacks, ECG changes that would be ignored in a healthy person take on a greater significance. First degree block, itself of no clinical importance, may point to intermittent complete block, and complete block is much more likely when the ECG of a currently asymptomatic patient shows second degree block. The ECGs in Figures 2.22, 2.23 and 2.24 are from patients with syncopal attacks, all of whom needed permanent pacemakers.

Left axis deviation usually indicates left anterior hemiblock, but a minor degree of left axis deviation with a narrow QRS complex can be accepted as a normal variant (Fig. 2.25). A QRS complex near the upper limit of the normal width with marked left axis deviation represents the full pattern of left anterior hemiblock (Fig. 2.26).

Second degree block (Wenckebach)

Note
- Sinus rhythm
- PR interval lengthens progressively from 360 ms to 440 ms and then a P wave is not conducted
- Small Q wave and inverted T wave in leads III and VF suggest an old inferior infarct

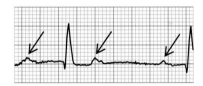

P waves

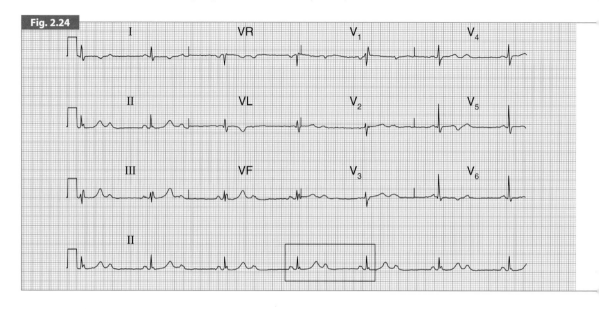

Fig. 2.24

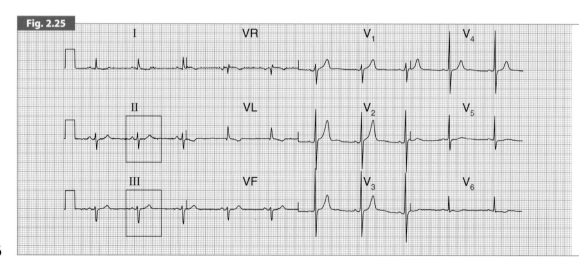

Fig. 2.25

Second degree block (2:1)

Note

- Sinus rhythm
- Alternate beats conducted and not conducted
- Lateral T wave inversion in leads I, VL, V_6 suggests ischaemia

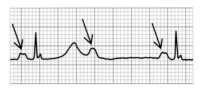

P waves

Left axis deviation

Note

- Sinus rhythm
- Dominant S waves in leads II and III: left axis deviation
- Normal QRS complex duration
- Lateral T wave inversion

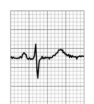 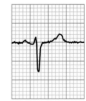

Dominant S waves in leads II and III

87

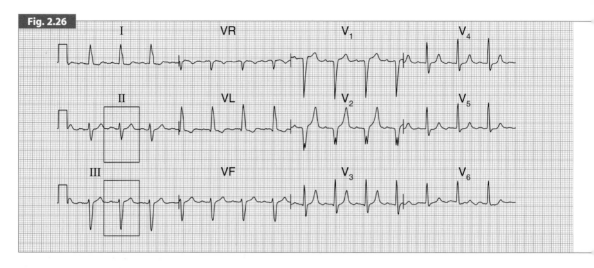

Fig. 2.26

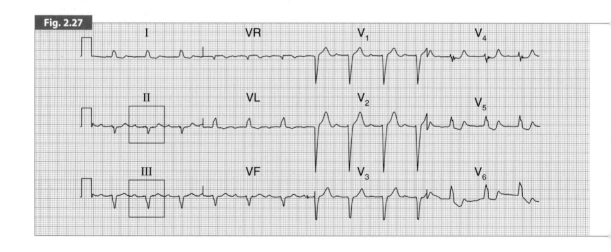

Fig. 2.27

Left anterior hemiblock

Note
- Sinus rhythm
- Left axis deviation
- Broad QRS complexes (122 ms)
- Inverted T waves in lead VL

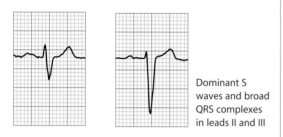

Dominant S waves and broad QRS complexes in leads II and III

First degree block and left bundle branch block (LBBB)

Note
- Sinus rhythm
- PR interval 300 ms
- LBBB pattern
- Broad QRS complexes

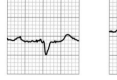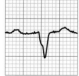

Long PR interval in leads II and III

Combinations of conduction abnormalities

ECG evidence of atrioventricular conduction abnormalities will not be associated with syncope unless there is intermittent second or third degree heart block with a bradycardia. It is, however, important to recognize the clinically less common conduction defects because they may be pointers to the cause of syncopal attacks.

When first degree block is associated with left bundle branch block (Fig. 2.27), conduction must be delayed in either the AV node, the His bundle or the right bundle branch as well as in the left bundle branch. The combination of first degree block and right bundle branch block (RBBB) (Fig. 2.28) shows that conduction has failed in the right bundle branch and is also beginning to fail elsewhere.

A combination of left anterior hemiblock and RBBB means that conduction into the ventricles is only passing through the posterior fascicle of the left bundle branch (Fig. 2.29). This is called 'bifascicular block'.

A combination of left anterior hemiblock, RBBB and first degree block suggests that there is disease in the remaining conducting pathway – either in the main His bundle or in the posterior fascicle of the left bundle branch. This is sometimes called 'trifascicular block' (Fig. 2.30). Complete conduction block in the right bundle and in both fascicles of the left bundle would, of course, cause complete (third degree) heart block.

Right axis deviation is not necessarily a feature of left posterior hemiblock, but, when combined with other evidence of conducting tissue disease such as first degree block (Fig. 2.31), it usually is.

A combination of second degree (2:1) block with left anterior hemiblock (Fig. 2.32) or with both left anterior hemiblock and RBBB (Fig. 2.33) suggests widespread conduction tissue disease.

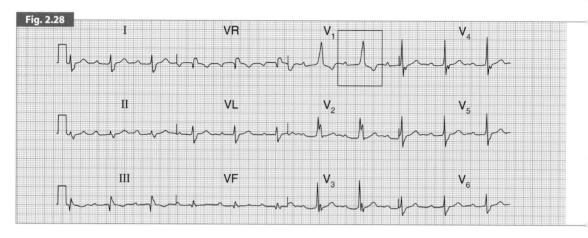

Fig. 2.28

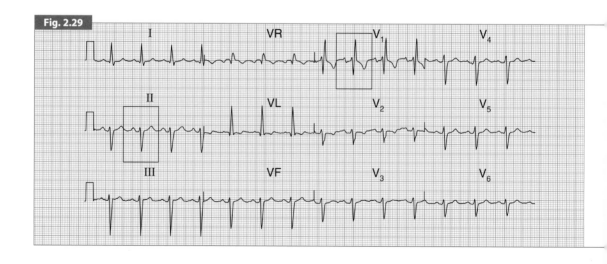

Fig. 2.29

First degree block and right bundle branch block (RBBB)

Note
- Sinus rhythm
- PR interval 328 ms
- Right axis deviation
- Broad QRS complexes
- RBBB pattern

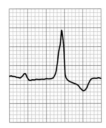

Long PR interval and RBBB pattern in lead V₁

Bifascicular block

Note
- Sinus rhythm
- PR interval normal (176 ms)
- Left anterior hemiblock
- RBBB

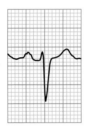 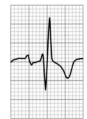

Left axis deviation and broad QRS complex in lead II

RBBB in lead V₁

91

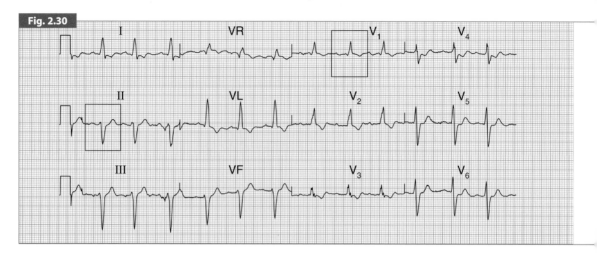

Fig. 2.30

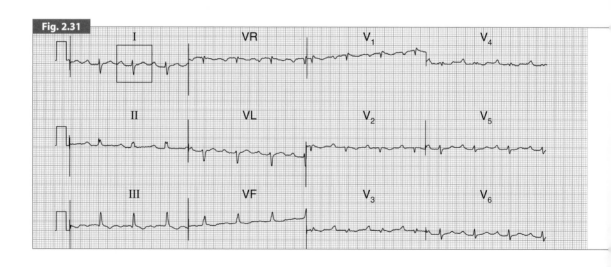

Fig. 2.31

Trifascicular block

Note
- Sinus rhythm
- PR interval 224 ms
- Left anterior hemiblock
- RBBB

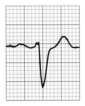
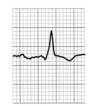

Left axis deviation
in lead II

RBBB in lead V$_1$

Left posterior hemiblock

Note
- Sinus rhythm
- First degree block (PR interval 320 ms)
- Right axis deviation
- This could represent right ventricular hypertrophy, but there is no dominant R wave in lead V$_1$

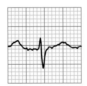

Long PR interval and deep S wave in lead I

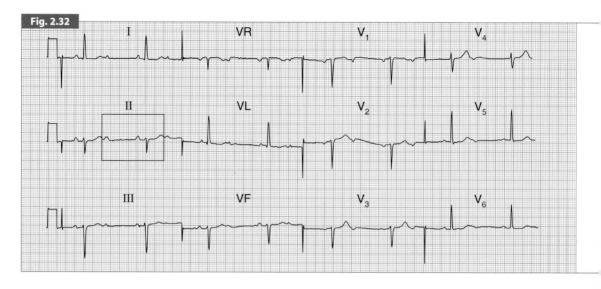

Fig. 2.32

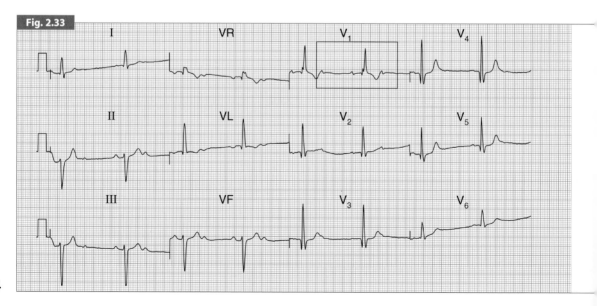

Fig. 2.33

Second degree block and left anterior hemiblock

Note
- Sinus rhythm
- Second degree block (2:1 type)
- Left anterior hemiblock
- Poor R wave progression suggests possible old anterior infarct

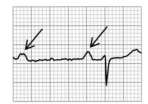

P waves in lead II

Second degree block, left anterior hemiblock and right bundle branch block (RBBB)

Note
- Sinus rhythm
- Second degree block (2:1 type)
- Left anterior hemiblock
- RBBB

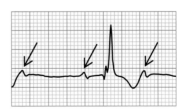

P waves and RBBB in lead V₁

95

AMBULATORY ECG RECORDING

The only way to be certain that a patient's symptoms are due to an arrhythmia is to show that an arrhythmia is present at the time of the symptoms. If symptoms occur frequently – say two or three times a week – a 24-h tape recording (called a 'Holter' record after its inventor) may show the abnormality. When symptoms are infrequent 'event recorders' are more useful, and these can either be patient-activated or programmed to detect rate or rhythm changes. Table 2.4 shows examples of these devices, and some of their advantages and disadvantages.

Figures 2.34, 2.35 and 2.36 show examples of ambulatory records obtained from patients who complained of syncopal attacks, but whose hearts were in sinus rhythm at the time they were first seen.

When an ambulatory record shows arrhythmias which are not accompanied by symptoms, it is difficult to be certain of their significance. When 24-h recordings are made from healthy volunteers, extrasystoles are found in about two-thirds of them, and a few will even show the R on T phenomenon. Episodes of supraventricular tachycardia are seen in about 3% of apparently healthy subjects, and ventricular tachycardia in about 1%.

If an ECG can be recorded at the time when the patient has symptoms, then there can be little doubt about the relationship between the symptoms and the cardiac rhythm, and the next two chapters deal with ECGs that may be recorded when a patient has either a tachycardia or a bradycardia.

Fig. 2.34

Ventricular tachycardia

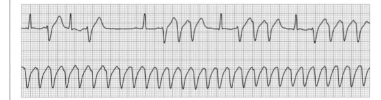

Note
- Ambulatory recording
- Initially sinus rhythm with ventricular extrasystoles
- Then salvos (three beats) of extrasystoles, leading to a broad complex tachycardia
- The change in the QRS complex configuration suggests that the tachycardia is ventricular, but a 12-lead ECG would be necessary to be certain

Fig. 2.35

Ventricular standstill

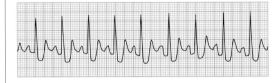

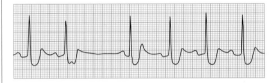

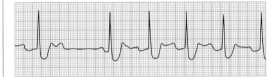

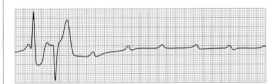

Note
- Ambulatory recording
- Top strip shows sinus rhythm with normal AV conduction
- Second strip shows SA block, which was asymptomatic
- Third strip shows second degree block, which was also asymptomatic
- Bottom strip shows a ventricular extrasystole followed by ventricular standstill. The patient lost consciousness due to this Stokes–Adams attack

Table 2.4 Ambulatory cardiac monitoring devices

Monitoring device		Mode of use
Holter monitor 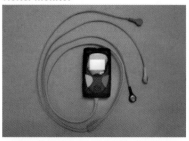	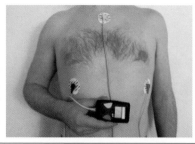	Usually three electrodes placed on chest wall for maximal signal; activation button can be used in association with patient diary to highlight symptomatic events
Cardiac memo 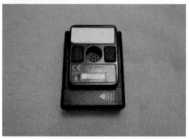	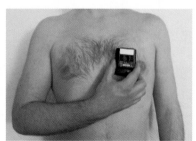	Device placed directly on to the skin by patient when symptomatic, or can be adapted to use with electrodes; traces can be downloaded by telephone
Loop recorder 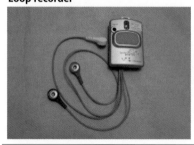	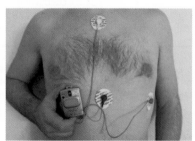	Usually three electrodes placed on chest wall; position of electrodes may require rotation, especially if there is skin reaction
Implantable loop recorder 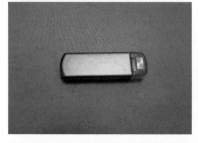	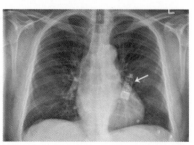	Requires subcutaneous implantation, a procedure taking around 20 min and with a low risk of infection Can be patient-activated

Duration and mode of recording	Applications	Comments
Usually 24 h, but up to 7 days Usually 1–2 channels, but up to 12 leads possible	Suitable for palpitations, syncope or presyncope occurring fairly frequently (e.g. daily)	Analysis time-consuming, but aided by software
10–20 recordings of 30–60 s	Suitable for palpitations lasting for several minutes, enabling patient to apply device and record trace	Not suitable for syncope, because patient activation required
Recording period programmable; usually 4 min pre- and post-activation Can record 2000–3000 periods ('loops') of ECG records, including patient-activated and autoactivated episodes Autoactivation function programmable, based on heart rate and on QRS complex duration and irregularity	Increasingly replacing memo devices Useful for diagnosis of palpitations or syncope	Can be kept in place for long periods, although batteries may need replacing periodically
Highly programmable; autoactivation can be based on heart rate and on QRS complex duration and irregularity	Especially useful for the diagnosis of rare rhythm disturbances and syncope	Orientation and site of implantation can be optimized prior to implantation Up to 14 months' battery life Surgical removal needed

Fig. 2.36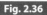

Sudden death due to ventricular fibrillation

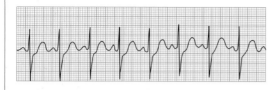

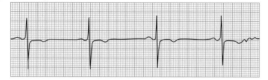

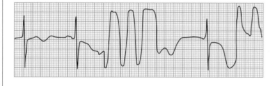

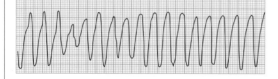

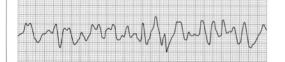

Note
- Ambulatory recording
- First strip shows sinus rhythm
- Sinus bradycardia then develops, with inversion of the T wave suggesting ischaemia
- Short runs of ventricular tachycardia (VT) lead to polymorphic VT
- Ventricular fibrillation then develops

The ECG when the patient has a tachycardia

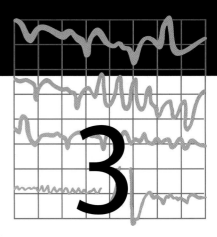

Mechanism of tachycardias	**102**
Enhanced automaticity and triggered activity	102
Abnormalities of cardiac rhythm due to re-entry	105
Differentiation between re-entry and enhanced automaticity	111
Tachycardias with symptoms	**113**
Sinus rhythm causing symptoms	113
Extrasystoles causing symptoms	115
Narrow complex tachycardias causing symptoms	117
Broad complex tachycardias causing symptoms	126
Special forms of ventricular tachycardia in patients with symptoms	144

Tachycardias associated with the Wolff–Parkinson–White syndrome	147
Management of arrhythmias	**150**
What to do when an arrhythmia is suspected	150
What to do when an arrhythmia is recorded	150
Extrasystoles	152
Sinus tachycardia	154
Atrial tachycardia	154
Atrioventricular nodal re-entry tachycardia (AVNRT, junctional tachycardia)	154
Atrial fibrillation and flutter	154
Ventricular tachycardia	155
The Wolff–Parkinson–White syndrome	155

Electrophysiology and catheter ablation	**155**
The endocardial ECG	156
Catheter ablation	157
Arrhythmias amenable to ablation	158
Indications for electrophysiology	162

Cardiac arrest	**162**
Management of cardiac arrest	164
Causes of cardiac arrest	165
Implanted cardioverter defibrillator (ICD) devices	165

The only tachycardia that can be (reasonably) reliably diagnosed from the patient's history is sinus tachycardia. A patient may notice the irregularity of atrial fibrillation, but it is easy to confuse this with multiple extrasystoles. The heart rate may give a clue to the nature of the arrhythmia (Table 3.1) but there is really no substitute for the ECG.

MECHANISM OF TACHYCARDIAS

Electrophysiology is the process of recording the ECG from inside the heart, using electrodes inserted via a peripheral vein. This is a highly specialized area, and yields additional information to that obtained from a conventional 12-lead ECG.

The main purpose of electrophysiological studies is to identify the site of origin of an arrhythmia. Arrhythmias occur either because of an abnormality of focal depolarization of the heart, or because of re-entry circuits. If the origin can be localized, the arrhythmia may be prevented permanently by ablation. This technique uses local endocardial (or more rarely epicardial) cautery burns to abolish areas of abnormal cardiac electrical activity, or to interrupt re-entry circuits.

Before the advent of electrical (ablation) therapy, the cause of arrhythmias was a fairly esoteric subject. Now, however, it is essential to understand the underlying electrical mechanisms, because they form the basis of ablation therapy.

ENHANCED AUTOMATICITY AND TRIGGERED ACTIVITY

If the intrinsic frequency of depolarization of the atrial, junctional or ventricular conducting tissue is increased, an abnormal rhythm may occur. This phenomenon is called 'enhanced automaticity'. Single early beats, or extrasystoles, may be due to enhanced automaticity arising from a myocardial focus. The most common example of a sustained rhythm due to enhanced automaticity is 'accelerated idioventricular rhythm', which is common after acute myocardial infarction. The ECG appearance (Fig. 3.1) resembles that of a slow ventricular tachycardia, and that is the old-fashioned name for this condition. This rhythm causes no symptoms, and should not be treated.

If the junctional intrinsic frequency is increased to a point at which it approximates to that of the SA node, an 'accelerated idionodal rhythm' results. This may appear to 'overtake' the P waves (Fig. 3.2). This rhythm used to be called a 'wandering pacemaker'. The term 'focal junctional tachycardia' is used in the (probably rare) instances of a supraventricular tachycardia originating around the AV node, by mechanisms other than re-entry.

Enhanced automaticity is also thought to be the mechanism causing some non-paroxysmal tachycardias, particularly those due to digoxin intoxication.

Table 3.1 **Physical signs and arrhythmias**

Pulse	Heart rate (beats/min)	Possible nature of any arrhythmia
Arterial pulse		
Regular	< 50	Sinus bradycardia
		Second or third degree block
		Atrial flutter with 3:1 or 4:1 block
		Idionodal rhythm (junctional escape), with or without sick sinus syndrome
	60–140	Probable sinus rhythm
	140–160	Sinus tachycardia or an arrhythmia
	150	Probable atrial flutter with 2:1 block
	140–170	Atrial tachycardia
		Atrioventricular re-entry tachycardia (AVRT)
		Atrioventricular nodal re-entry tachycardia (AVNRT; junctional (nodal) tachycardia)
		Ventricular tachycardia
	> 180	Probable ventricular tachycardia
	300	Atrial flutter with 1:1 conduction
Irregular		Marked sinus arrhythmia
		Extrasystoles (supraventricular or ventricular)
		Atrial fibrillation
		Atrial flutter with variable block
		Rhythm varying between sinus rhythm and any arrhythmia or conduction defect
Jugular venous pulse		
More pulsations visible than heart rate		Second or third degree block
		Cannon waves – third degree block

 Fig. 3.1

Accelerated idioventricular rhythm

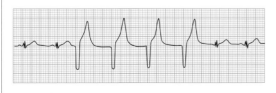

Note
- After two sinus beats, there are four beats of ventricular origin with a rate of 75/min
- Sinus rhythm is then restored

103

Fig. 3.2

Accelerated idionodal rhythm

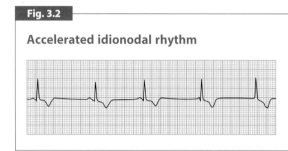

Note
- After three sinus beats, the sinus rate slows slightly
- A nodal rhythm appears and 'overtakes' the P waves

Fig. 3.3

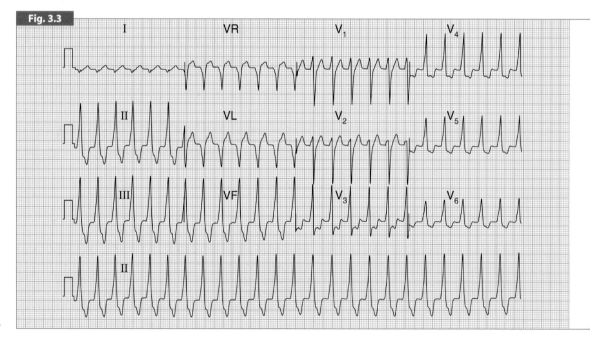

Fig. 3.4

Re-entry pathways in the pre-excitation syndromes

The Wolff–Parkinson–White syndrome type A

The Lown–Ganong–Levine syndrome

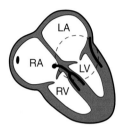

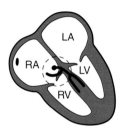

Note
- Broken lines indicate the potential re-entry pathways in AVRT

Right ventricular outflow tract ventricular tachycardia (RVOT-VT)

Note
- Broad complex tachycardia
- Left bundle branch block and right axis deviation, typical of RVOT-VT

'Triggered activity' results from late depolarizations which occur after normal depolarization, during what would normally be a period of repolarization. Like enhanced automaticity, this can cause extrasystoles or a sustained arrhythmia, such as right ventricular outflow tract ventricular tachycardia (RVOT-VT) (Fig. 3.3).

ABNORMALITIES OF CARDIAC RHYTHM DUE TO RE-ENTRY

Normal conduction results in the uniform spread of the depolarization wave front in a constant direction. Should the direction of depolarization be reversed in some part of the heart, such as in an accessory connection between the atria and ventricles, it becomes possible for a circular or 're-entry' pathway to be set up. Activation travels round and round the circuit, causing a tachycardia such as the atrioventricular re-entry tachycardia (AVRT) experienced by patients with the Wolff–Parkinson–White (WPW) syndrome or the Lown–Ganong–Levine (LGL) syndrome (Fig. 3.4). **105**

ATRIOVENTRICULAR RE-ENTRY TACHYCARDIA (AVRT)

In the pre-excitation syndromes, normal and accessory pathways between an atrium and a ventricle together form an anatomical circuit round which depolarization can reverberate, causing a 're-entry' tachycardia (Fig. 3.5). Once established, a circular wave of depolarization will continue until some part of the pathway fails to conduct. Alternatively, the circular wave may be interrupted by the arrival of another depolarization wave, set up by an ectopic focus (e.g. an extrasystole).

In the WPW syndrome, the re-entry circuit comprises the normal AV node–His bundle connection between the atria and the ventricles, and an accessory pathway, the bundle of Kent, which also connects the atria and ventricles, bypassing the AV node (Fig. 3.4). If forward conduction in the accessory pathway is blocked, depolarization can spread down the normal pathway and back (i.e. retrogradely) via the accessory pathway, to reactivate the atria. Recurrent activation of the circuit can cause a 'circus movement', resulting in a 'reciprocating tachycardia'.

The tachycardia is described as 'orthodromic' when conduction within the His bundle is in the normal direction: the ECG then has narrow QRS complexes, and sometimes P waves are visible just after each QRS complex. Less commonly, depolarization passes down the accessory pathway and retrogradely up the His bundle, to cause an 'antidromic reciprocating tachycardia', in which the QRS complexes are broad

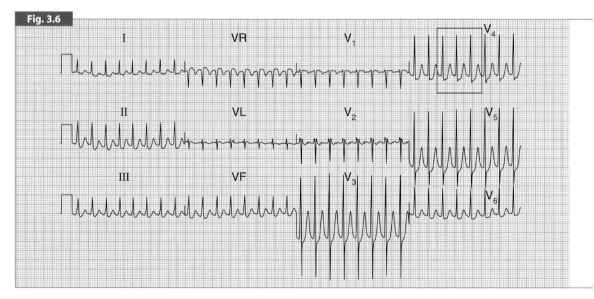

Fig. 3.6

Fig. 3.5

Re-entry mechanisms causing tachycardia

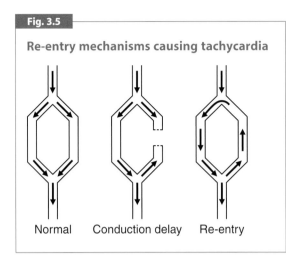

Normal   Conduction delay   Re-entry

Supraventricular tachycardia

Note
- Narrow complex tachycardia
- No P waves visible
- Some ST segment depression, suggesting ischaemia

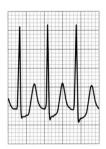

Narrow complexes with ST segment depression in lead V$_4$

and slurred, and P waves may or may not be seen. When the re-entry tachycardia is associated with a narrow QRS complex (i.e. when it is orthodromic), the pattern resembles a junctional (AV nodal re-entry) tachycardia (see below) and the presence of a pre-excitation syndrome may not be suspected (Figs 3.6 and 3.7).

The broad complex (antidromic reciprocating) tachycardias which occur in patients with the WPW syndrome may resemble ventricular tachycardia (Fig. 3.8). A very irregular broad complex tachycardia, as shown in the lower trace of Figure 3.8, will usually be due to the WPW syndrome with atrial fibrillation and antidromic conduction through the re-entry circuit. This rhythm can only be distinguished with certainty from atrial fibrillation and left bundle branch block if the appearance of the ECG in sinus rhythm is known. Superficially, the rhythm may resemble torsade de pointes ventricular tachycardia, but it lacks the characteristic 'writhing' of the QRS complexes that is associated with this arrhythmia.

ATRIAL TACHYCARDIA

Re-entry within the atrial muscle causes a tachycardia characterized by P waves with a shape different from that of those related to sinus rhythm. The PR interval is usually short (Fig. 3.9). Atrial tachycardia can also result from enhanced automaticity.

Fig. 3.7

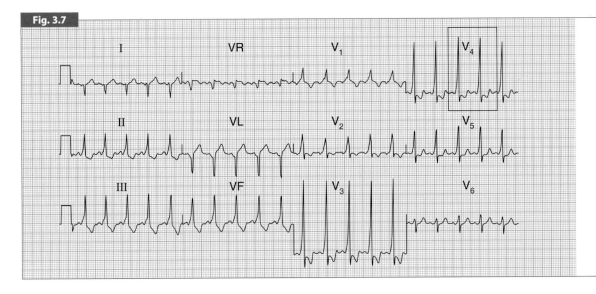

Fig. 3.8

Tachycardias in the Wolff–Parkinson–White syndrome

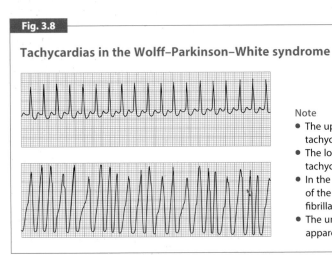

Note
- The upper trace shows a narrow complex (orthodromic) tachycardia
- The lower trace shows a wide complex (antidromic) tachycardia
- In the lower trace the marked irregularity and variation of the complexes suggest that the rhythm is atrial fibrillation
- The underlying diagnosis of the WPW syndrome is not apparent from either trace

Sinus rhythm, the Wolff–Parkinson–White syndrome, type A

Note
- Same patient as in Figure 3.6, after cardioversion
- Sinus rhythm
- Short PR interval
- Broad QRS complexes with delta wave
- Dominant R wave in lead V_1 shows the WPW syndrome type A

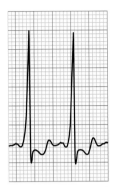

Short PR interval and delta wave in lead V_4

ATRIAL FLUTTER

Atrial flutter is an organized atrial rhythm with a rate of 250–350/min. This rhythm depends on a variety of re-entry circuits, which often occupy large areas of the atrium and are known as 'macro-re-entrant' circuits. The most common type of flutter, 'isthmus-dependent' flutter, involves circuits utilizing the cavotricuspid isthmus. The involvement of a defined isthmus is important in considering ablation therapy (see p. 157).

AV NODAL RE-ENTRY TACHYCARDIA (AVNRT)

Atrioventricular nodal re-entry tachycardia (AVNRT), also known as atrioventricular nodal reciprocating tachycardia, originates in the AV node or His bundle. It may be facilitated by a congenital abnormality of the AV node, in which there are two (or sometimes more) electrically distinct pathways. These allow re-entry to start and be sustained within the node itself. In the absence of a tachycardia, the ECG has no distinguishing features, so the potential for an AVNRT cannot be detected from the ECG, unlike in cases of the WPW and LGL syndromes. During AVNRT, atrial and ventricular activation are virtually simultaneous, so the P wave is hidden within the QRS complex (Fig. 3.10). AVNRT used to be called 'junctional tachycardia'.

VENTRICULAR TACHYCARDIA

Ventricular tachycardia may be due to re-entry through circuits within the ventricles (for example around areas of scar tissue following myocardial infarction), or may result from enhanced automaticity or triggered activity. The broad QRS complexes are of a constant configuration and are fairly regular if the re-entry pathway is constant (Fig. 3.11).

109

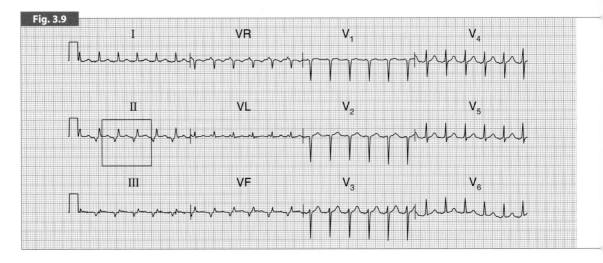

Fig. 3.9

Fig. 3.10

AV nodal re-entry tachycardia (AVNRT)

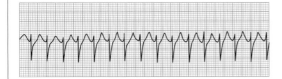

Note
- No P waves can be seen
- QRS complexes are narrow, and completely regular at 165/min

Fig. 3.11

Ventricular tachycardia

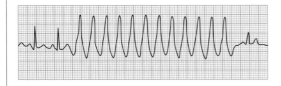

Note
- Two sinus beats are followed by ventricular tachycardia at 200/min
- The complexes are regular, with little variation in shape
- Sinus rhythm is then restored

Atrial tachycardia

Note
- P waves visible, but they are inverted in several leads
- Rate 140/min
- Normal QRS complexes

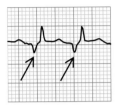

Inverted P waves in lead II

DIFFERENTIATION BETWEEN RE-ENTRY AND ENHANCED AUTOMATICITY

Except in the case of the pre-excitation syndromes, there is no certain way of distinguishing from the surface ECG between a tachycardia due to enhanced automaticity and one due to re-entry. In general, however, tachycardias that follow or are terminated by extrasystoles, and those that can be initiated or inhibited by appropriately timed intracardiac pacing impulses, are likely to be due to re-entry (Figs 3.12 and 3.13).

The differentiation between tachycardias caused by enhanced automaticity and those caused by re-entry does not affect the choice of drug treatment, and both can be treated by ablation.

Fig. 3.12

Atrial tachycardia

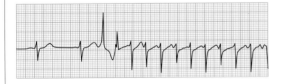

Note
- After two sinus beats there is one ventricular extrasystole, and then a narrow complex that is probably supraventricular
- Atrial tachycardia is induced
- P waves are visible at the end of the T wave of the preceding beat

---

Fig. 3.13

AV nodal re-entry tachycardia (AVNRT)

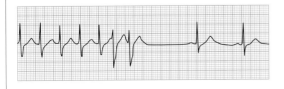

Note
- Five beats of AVNRT at 143/min are followed by two ventricular extrasystoles
- These interrupt the tachycardia, and sinus rhythm is restored

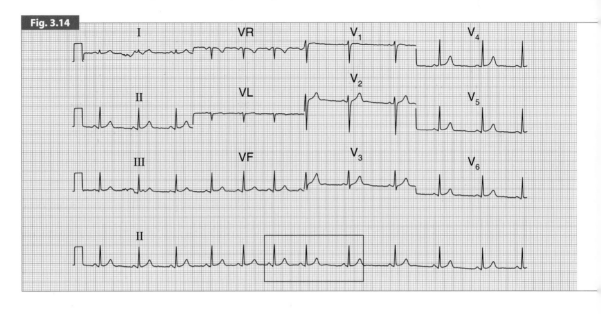

Fig. 3.14

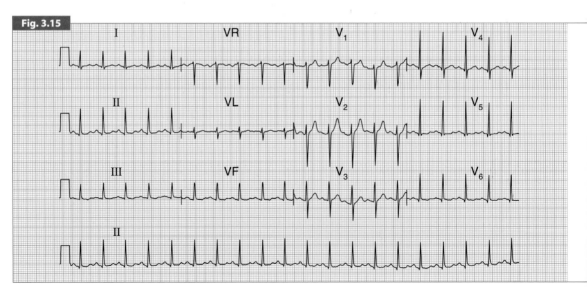

Fig. 3.15

Sinus arrhythmia

Note
- Sinus rhythm
- All P waves identical
- Progressive shortening then lengthening of the R–R interval

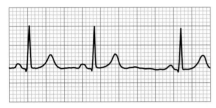

Identical P waves and irregular R–R interval

Sinus tachycardia

Note
- Sinus rhythm, rate 120/min
- Nonspecific ST segment changes in leads III, VF, V$_6$

TACHYCARDIAS WITH SYMPTOMS

SINUS RHYTHM CAUSING SYMPTOMS

Sinus rhythm can be irregular (sinus arrhythmia) but the patient is never aware of this. The ECG of a patient with sinus arrhythmia (Fig. 3.14) may suggest atrial extrasystoles – but in sinus rhythm, P wave morphology is constant while with atrial extrasystoles it varies.

Patients often complain of palpitations that are due to sinus tachycardia: the main causes are exercise, anxiety, thyrotoxicosis and the treatment of asthma with beta-adrenergic agonists, and other causes are summarized in Box 1.1 (p. 3). The ECG in Figure 3.15 shows sinus tachycardia due to an unusual cause – the habitual drinking of large quantities of cola.

When sinus tachycardia results from anxiety, heart rates of up to 150/min are possible and the rhythm may be mistaken for an atrial tachycardia. Pressure on the carotid sinus will cause transient slowing of the heart rate and the P waves will become more obvious (see Fig. 3.53, p. 153).

Fig. 3.16

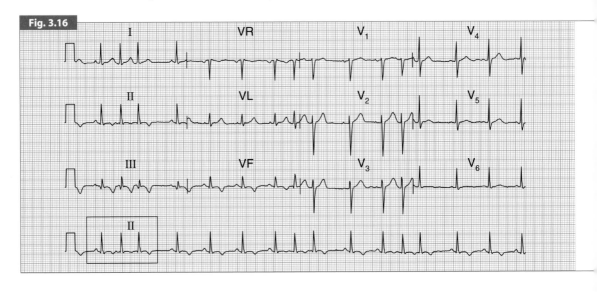

Fig. 3.17

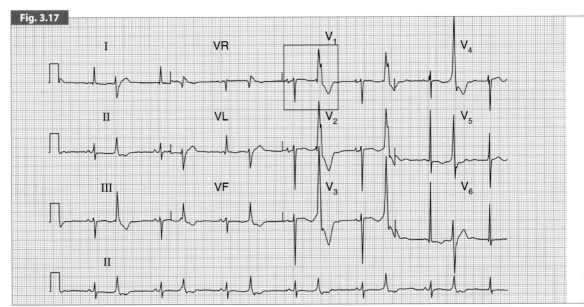

Supraventricular extrasystoles
Note
- Sinus rhythm with atrial and junctional extrasystoles
- Normal axis
- Normal QRS complexes
- Inverted T waves in leads III, VF

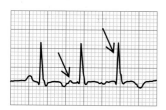

First beat: normal; second beat: atrial extrasystole, with abnormal P wave; third beat: AV nodal (junctional) extrasystole, with no P wave

EXTRASYSTOLES CAUSING SYMPTOMS

An ECG is necessary to differentiate between supraventricular and ventricular extrasystoles.

When extrasystoles have a supraventricular origin (Fig. 3.16), the QRS complex is narrow and both it and the T wave have the same configuration as in the sinus beat. Atrial extrasystoles have abnormal P waves. Junctional (AV nodal) extrasystoles either have a P wave very close to the QRS complex (in front of it or behind it) or have no visible P waves.

Ventricular extrasystoles produce wide QRS complexes of abnormal shape, and the T wave is also usually abnormal. No P waves are present (Fig. 3.17).

When a ventricular extrasystole appears on the upstroke of the preceding beat, the 'R on T' phenomenon is said to be present (Fig. 3.18). This can initiate ventricular fibrillation, but usually it does not do so.

Ventricular extrasystoles
Note
- Sinus rhythm with coupled ventricular extrasystoles
- Sinus beats show tall R waves and inverted T waves in leads V_5–V_6 (indicating left ventricular hypertrophy)
- Extrasystoles are of right bundle branch block (RBBB) configuration, and their T wave inversion has no other significance

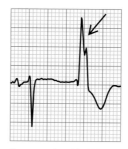

Extrasystole with RBBB configuration in lead V_1

115

Fig. 3.18

R on T phenomenon

Note

• Ventricular extrasystoles occurring near the peak of the preceding T wave

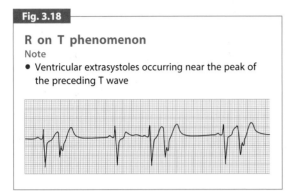

Box 3.1 Narrow complex tachycardias

A regular narrow complex tachycardia may be:
• Sinus rhythm
• Atrial tachycardia
• Atrial flutter
• AV nodal re-entry tachycardia (AVNRT) – the commonest type of supraventricular tachycardia
• AV re-entry tachycardia (AVRT), caused by the WPW syndrome with orthodromic conduction through the AV node–His bundle pathway

An irregular narrow complex tachycardia is usually:
• Atrial fibrillation

Fig. 3.19

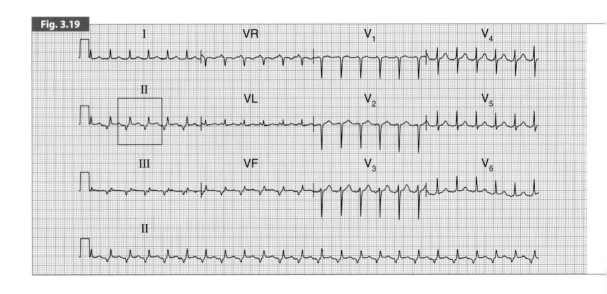

NARROW COMPLEX TACHYCARDIAS CAUSING SYMPTOMS

A tachycardia can be described as 'narrow complex' if the QRS complex is of normal duration, i.e. < 120 ms. Although sinus, atrial and junctional arrhythmias are all supraventricular, the term 'supraventricular tachycardia' is often inappropriately used interchangeably with junctional or atrioventricular nodal re-entry tachycardia (AVNRT). All these supraventricular rhythms have QRS complexes of normal shape and width, and the T waves have the same shape as in the sinus beat.

Types of narrow complex tachycardias are listed in Box 3.1.

ATRIAL TACHYCARDIA

In atrial tachycardia (Fig. 3.19), P waves are present but they have an abnormal shape. They are sometimes hidden in the T wave of the preceding beat.

The P wave rate is in the range 130–250/min. When the atrial rate exceeds about 180/min, physiological block will occur in the AV node, so that the ventricular rate becomes half that of the atria. Atrial tachycardia with 2:1 block is characteristic of (but not commonly seen with) digoxin toxicity.

ATRIAL FLUTTER

In atrial flutter, the atrial rate is 300/min and the P waves form a continuous 'sawtooth' pattern. As the AV node usually fails to conduct all the P waves, the relationship between P waves and QRS complexes is usually 2:1, 3:1 or 4:1. Figure 3.20 shows atrial flutter with 2:1 block, giving a ventricular rate of 150/min. The ECG in Figure 3.21 is from the same patient after reversion to sinus rhythm.

The ECG in Figure 3.22 shows atrial flutter with 4:1 block.

The ECG in Figure 3.23 shows a narrow complex (and therefore supraventricular) rhythm with a rate of 300/min. This is almost certainly atrial flutter with 1:1 conduction.

If the ventricular rate is rapid and P waves cannot be seen, carotid sinus pressure will usually increase the block in the AV node and make the 'sawtooth' more obvious (see Fig. 3.54, p. 153).

Atrial tachycardia

Note

- Narrow complex tachycardia, heart rate 140/min
- Abnormally shaped P waves, one per QRS complex
- Short PR interval
- ECG otherwise normal

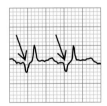

Abnormal P waves in lead II

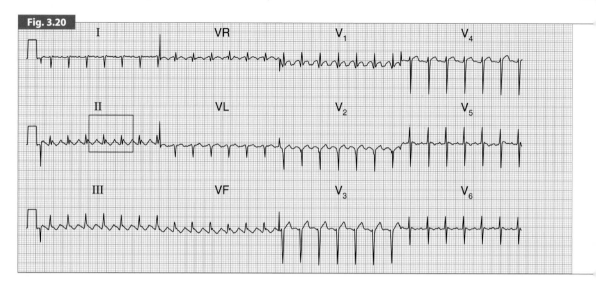

Fig. 3.20

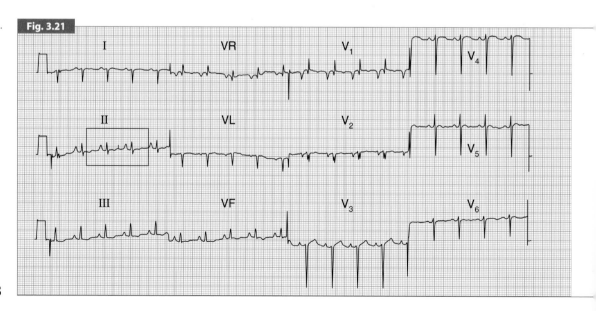

Fig. 3.21

Atrial flutter with 2:1 block

Note
- Regular narrow complex tachycardia
- 'Sawtooth' of atrial flutter most easily seen in lead II

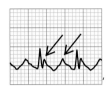

Flutter waves in lead II

Sinus rhythm, following cardioversion

Note
- Same patient as in Figure 3.20
- Sinus rhythm
- Right axis deviation
- Dominant R waves in lead V_1
- Deep S waves in lead V_6, suggesting right ventricular hypertrophy
- The cardiac axis and QRS complexes have not been changed by cardioversion

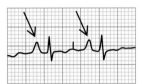

P waves in lead II

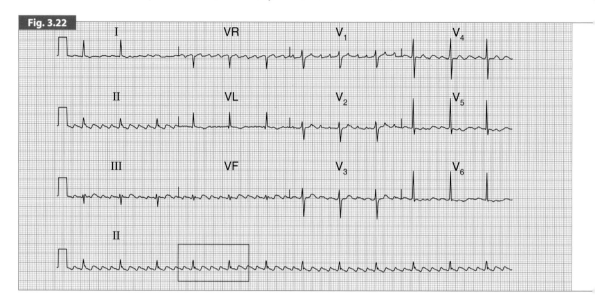

Fig. 3.22

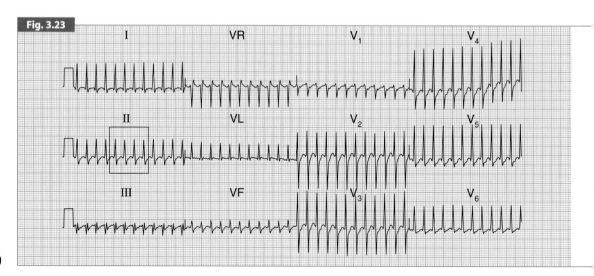

Fig. 3.23

Atrial flutter with 4:1 block

Note

- With 4:1 block and a ventricular rate of 72/min, flutter waves can be seen in all leads

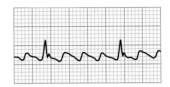

Flutter waves

Atrial flutter with 1:1 conduction

Note

- Narrow complex tachycardia at nearly 300/min
- No P waves visible
- Ventricular rate suggests that the underlying rhythm is atrial flutter

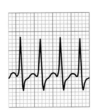

Narrow complex tachycardia at 300/min in lead II

Fig. 3.24

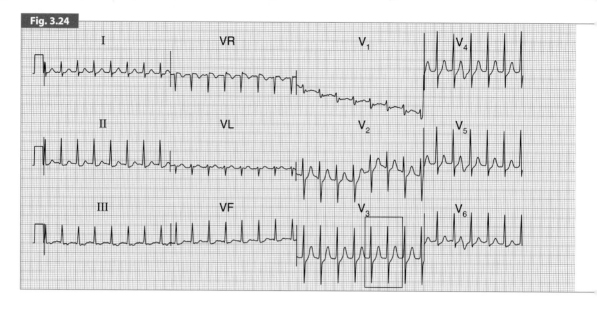

Fig. 3.25

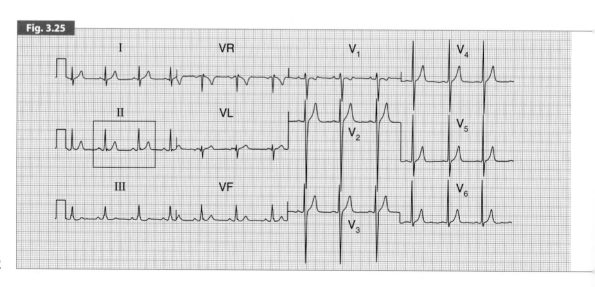

Atrioventricular nodal re-entry tachycardia (AVNRT)

Note
- Regular narrow complex tachycardia, rate 150/min
- No P waves visible
- ST segment depression in leads II–III, VF suggests ischaemia

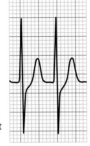

Narrow complexes at about 150/min in lead V₃

ATRIOVENTRICULAR NODAL RE-ENTRY TACHYCARDIA (AVNRT) OR 'JUNCTIONAL' TACHYCARDIA

In AVNRT, no P waves can be seen (Fig. 3.10, p. 110). Carotid sinus pressure either reverts the heart to sinus rhythm or has no effect (see Fig. 3.55, p. 153).

The ECG in Figure 3.24 shows a narrow complex tachycardia at 150/min, without any obvious P waves. After reversion to sinus rhythm (Fig. 3.25), the shape of the QRS complexes does not change.

The ECG in Figure 3.6 (p. 106) shows what appears to be a straightforward AVNRT, but on return to sinus rhythm (Fig. 3.7) it shows the Wolff–Parkinson–White type A pattern. The tachycardia was therefore orthodromic, with the re-entry circuit involving anterograde (normal) conduction down the AV node and His bundle (see Fig. 3.5, p. 107).

Sinus rhythm following cardioversion

Note
- Same patient as in Figure 3.24
- Sinus rhythm
- QRS complexes and T waves are the same shape as in AVNRT (Fig. 3.24)
- Now no suggestion of ischaemia

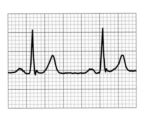

Sinus rhythm

Fig. 3.26

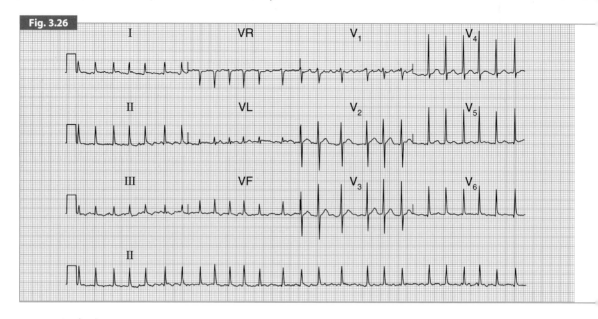

Fig. 3.27

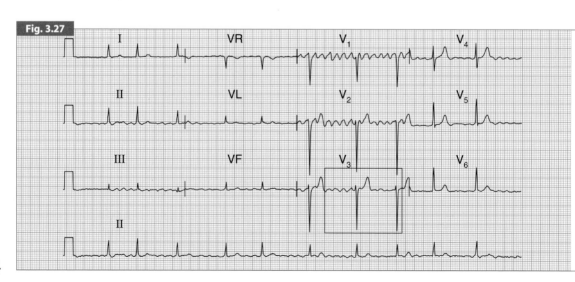

Atrial fibrillation

Note
- Irregular narrow complex tachycardia, 150/min
- During long R–R intervals, irregular baseline can be seen
- Suggestion of flutter waves in lead V₁

ATRIAL FIBRILLATION

In atrial fibrillation, disorganized atrial activity causes the P waves to disappear and the ECG baseline becomes totally irregular (Fig. 3.26). At times atrial activity may become sufficiently synchronized for a 'flutter-like' pattern to appear, but this rapidly breaks up (Fig. 3.27). In atrial fibrillation, as opposed to atrial flutter, the frequency of the QRS complexes is totally irregular.

Some causes of atrial fibrillation are summarized in Box 3.2.

Atrial fibrillation

Note
- Irregular narrow complex rhythm
- Apparent flutter waves in lead V₁, but these are not constant and from leads II and V₃ it is clear that this is atrial fibrillation

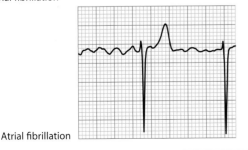

Atrial fibrillation

Box 3.2 Causes of atrial fibrillation (paroxysmal or persistent)

- Rheumatic heart disease
- Thyrotoxicosis
- Alcoholism
- Cardiomyopathy
- Acute myocardial infarction
- Chronic ischaemic heart disease
- Hypertension
- Myocarditis
- Pericarditis
- Pulmonary embolism
- Pneumonia
- Cardiac surgery
- The Wolff–Parkinson–White syndrome
- 'Lone' (i.e. no cause found)

BROAD COMPLEX TACHYCARDIAS CAUSING SYMPTOMS

'Broad complex' tachycardias are those in which the QRS complex duration exceeds 120 ms and which are not due to sinus rhythm with bundle branch block. Broad complex tachycardias can be either supraventricular with bundle branch block; or due to the Wolff–Parkinson–White syndrome; or may be ventricular in origin. The types of broad complex tachycardia are listed in Box 3.3.

A supraventricular origin for a broad complex tachycardia can only be diagnosed with certainty when there is intermittent sinus rhythm with the same QRS complex configuration as is seen in the tachycardia (Fig. 3.28).

Here we are concerned with broad complex rhythms without obvious P waves. These could be atrial fibrillation or junctional rhythms with bundle branch block, or could be ventricular rhythms. The differentiation of broad complex tachycardias can be difficult. It is not possible to distinguish between supraventricular and ventricular rhythms from the clinical state of the patient. Either type of rhythm can

Box 3.3 Broad complex tachycardias

- Any supraventricular rhythm with bundle branch block
- Accelerated idioventricular rhythm (rate < 120/min)
- Ventricular tachycardia
- Torsade de pointes ventricular tachycardia
- The Wolff–Parkinson–White (WPW) syndrome

An irregular broad complex tachycardia is likely to be:
- Atrial fibrillation with bundle branch block
- Atrial fibrillation with the WPW syndrome

Box 3.4 Causes of ventricular tachycardia

- Acute myocardial infarction
- Chronic ischaemia
- Cardiomyopathy:
  — hypertrophic
  — dilated
- Mitral valve prolapse
- Myocarditis
- Electrolyte imbalance
- Congenital long QT syndrome
- Drugs:
  — antiarrhythmic
  — digoxin
- Idiopathic

Fig. 3.28

Junctional tachycardia with bundle branch block

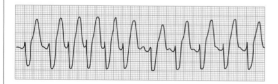

Note
- A single sinus beat with a broad QRS complex is followed by five beats without P waves, but with the same broad QRS complex pattern
- Sinus rhythm is then restored and the QRS complex remains unchanged
- The tachycardia must be supraventricular with bundle branch block

be well tolerated, and either can lead to cardiovascular collapse. However, broad complex tachycardias occurring in the course of an acute myocardial infarction (which is when they are most often seen) are almost always ventricular in origin. Other causes of ventricular tachycardia (VT) are listed in Box 3.4.

With these things in mind, the ECG should be analysed logically. Look in turn for the following features:

1. The presence of P waves. If there is one P wave per QRS complex, it must be sinus rhythm with bundle branch block. If P waves can be seen at a slower rate than the QRS complexes, it must be VT.
2. QRS complex duration. If longer than 160 ms, it is probably VT.
3. QRS complex regularity. VT is usually regular. An irregular broad complex tachycardia usually means atrial fibrillation with abnormal conduction.
4. The cardiac axis. VT is usually associated with left axis deviation.
5. QRS complex configuration. If the QRS complexes in the V leads all point either upwards or downwards ('concordance') it is probably VT.
6. When the QRS complex shows a right bundle branch block pattern, a supraventricular tachycardia with abnormal conduction is more likely if the second R peak is higher than the first. VT is likely if the first R peak is higher.
7. The presence of fusion and capture beats indicates that the broad complexes are due to VT (see p. 142).

P WAVES

The ECG in Figure 3.29 is from a patient with an acute infarction, and shows a broad complex rhythm at about 110/min. One P wave per QRS complex can clearly be seen, and this is obviously sinus rhythm with left bundle branch block (LBBB).

The ECG in Figure 3.30 shows a very irregular broad complex rhythm with no obvious P waves. There is an obvious LBBB pattern in leads V_5 and V_6. Whether the R–R interval is short or long, the appearance of the QRS complex is the same. The irregularity is the key to the diagnosis of atrial fibrillation with LBBB.

The ECG in Figure 3.31 is also an example of atrial fibrillation and LBBB, but this is not quite as obvious as in Figure 3.30. The QRS complexes at first sight may appear regular, but on close inspection they are not. The LBBB is also not so obvious, but can be seen in lead I.

Occasionally it may be possible to identify P waves with a slower rate than the QRS complexes, indicating that the QRS complexes must be ventricular in origin. A 12-lead ECG during the tachycardia is important for this, because P waves may be visible in some leads but not in others (Fig. 3.32).

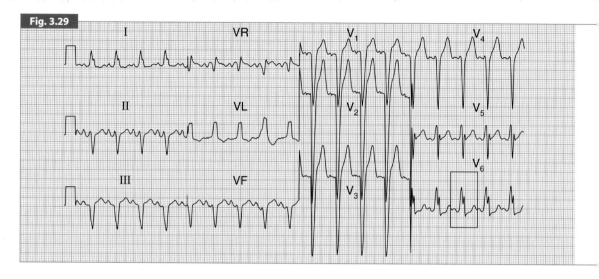

Fig. 3.29

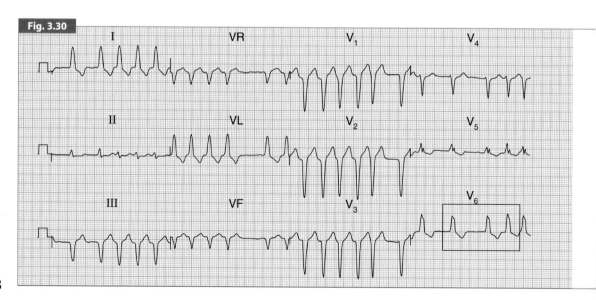

Fig. 3.30

Sinus rhythm with left bundle branch block (LBBB)

Note
- Sinus rhythm
- Left axis deviation
- Wide QRS complexes of LBBB configuration

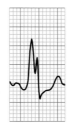

M wave of LBBB in lead V_6

Atrial fibrillation with left bundle branch block (LBBB)

Note
- Recorded at half sensitivity (0.5 cm = 1 mV)
- Irregular broad complex tachycardia
- No obvious P waves, but irregular baseline in lead VR
- LBBB configuration of QRS complexes

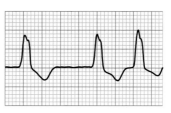

M wave of LBBB in lead V_6

Fig. 3.31

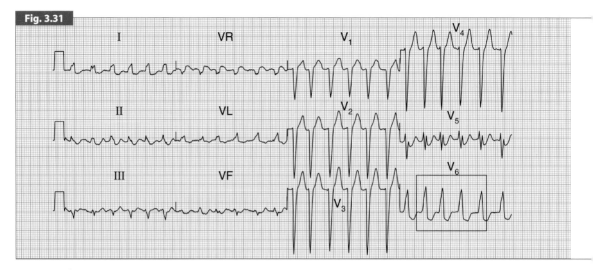

Fig. 3.32

Ventricular tachycardia

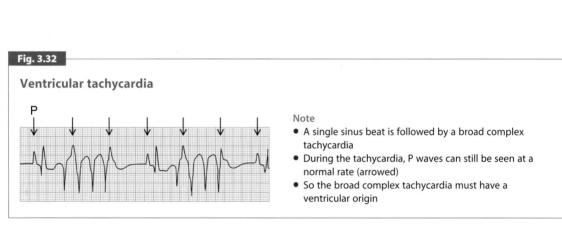

P

Note
- A single sinus beat is followed by a broad complex tachycardia
- During the tachycardia, P waves can still be seen at a normal rate (arrowed)
- So the broad complex tachycardia must have a ventricular origin

Atrial fibrillation with left bundle branch block (LBBB)

Note
- Broad complex rhythm at 140/min
- Slightly irregular rhythm, best seen in lead V_6
- LBBB pattern, most obvious in lead I

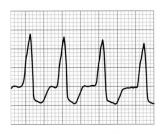

Irregular rhythm in lead V_6

THE QRS COMPLEX

The ECG in Figure 3.33 shows a broad complex tachycardia recorded from a patient with an acute infarction, and there is no question that this represents VT. The important features are:

- regular rhythm at 160/min (a fairly typical rate)
- very broad complexes of 360 ms duration (when the QRS complex duration is > 160 ms, VT is likely)
- left axis deviation
- in the V leads the QRS complexes all point in the same direction (in this case downwards). This is called 'concordance'.

The ECG in Figure 3.34 shows an ECG from another patient with an acute infarction. The shape of the QRS complexes is different from that in Figure 3.33, but the principles are the same:

- The rhythm is regular.
- The complexes are very broad.
- There is left axis deviation.
- The complexes show concordance.

The ECG in Figure 3.35 shows another example of VT, but this time the axis is normal. Unfortunately the 'rules' for diagnosing VT are not absolute and one or more of the features above may not be present.

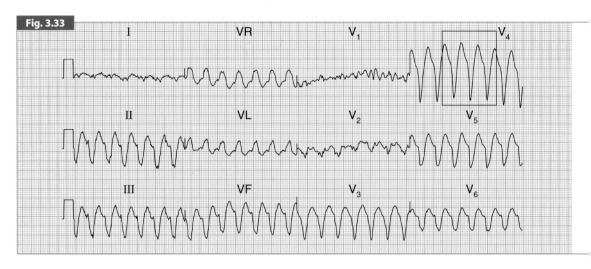

Fig. 3.33

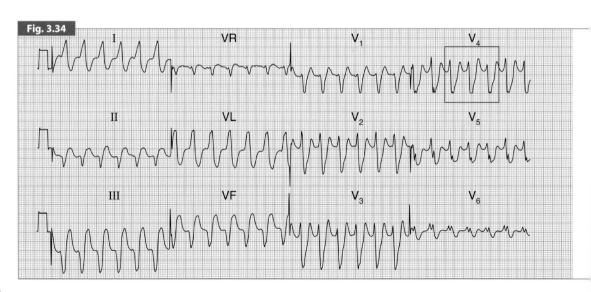

Fig. 3.34

Ventricular tachycardia

Note

- Regular broad complex tachycardia, 160/min
- Appearance of lead V₁ is clearly an artefact
- Left axis deviation
- All complexes in the chest leads point downwards (concordance)
- There are no R waves in the chest leads, so the complexes are sometimes known as 'QS' complexes

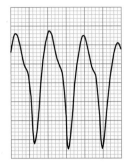

Broad complexes

Ventricular tachycardia

Note

- Regular broad complex tachycardia, 150/min
- No P waves visible
- Left axis deviation
- Concordance of QRS complexes in chest leads

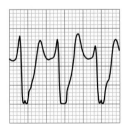

Broad complexes

Fig. 3.35

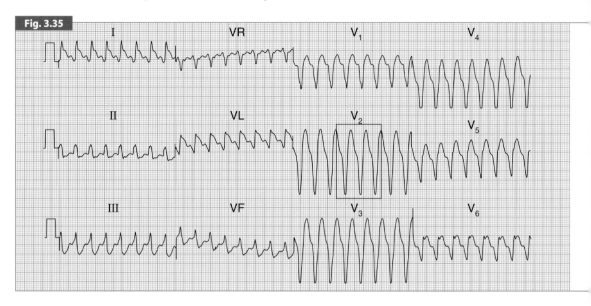

Fig. 3.36

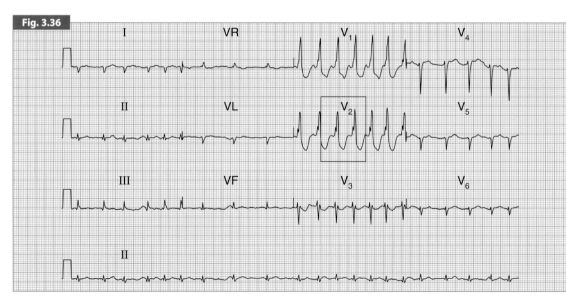

Ventricular tachycardia

Note

- Regular broad complex tachycardia
- No P waves
- Normal axis
- Concordance (downward) of QRS complexes in the chest leads

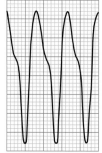

Broad complexes

Atrial fibrillation with right bundle branch block (RBBB)

Note

- Irregular broad complex tachycardia
- Right axis deviation
- QRS complexes show RBBB pattern, with second R peak higher than the first

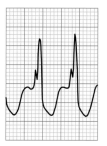

R^1 taller than R peak in lead V_2

The ECG in Figure 3.36 shows atrial fibrillation with an abnormal QRS complex, the duration of which (116 ms) is just within the normal range. The RSR^1 pattern, most obviously seen in lead V_2, and the slurred S wave in lead V_6, show that this is partial right bundle branch block (RBBB). Note that the second R peak of the QRS complex (R^1) is higher than first peak. This is characteristic of RBBB. These features show that this is a supraventricular rhythm.

The ECG in Figure 3.37 shows a regular tachycardia with no P waves and a QRS complex showing an RBBB pattern. The duration of the QRS complex is at the upper limit of normal, at 120 ms. This might be a supraventricular tachycardia (probably AVNRT) with RBBB conduction, or it might be a fascicular tachycardia. A fascicular tachycardia usually arises in the posterior fascicle of the left bundle branch. Typically there is left axis deviation (not present here). Fascicular tachycardia is an unusual rhythm with a benign prognosis, and it typically responds to verapamil.

The ECG in Figure 3.38 shows how difficult differentiation between supraventricular and ventricular rhythms can be. Some features suggest a supraventricular, and some a ventricular, origin of the rhythm.

135

Fig. 3.37

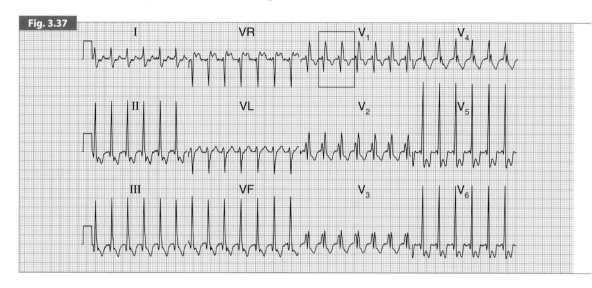

Fig. 3.38

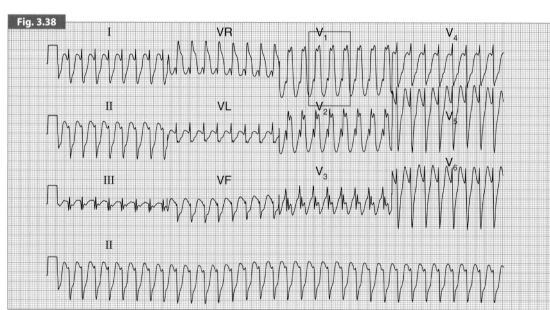

?Junctional tachycardia with right bundle branch block or ?fascicular tachycardia

Note
- Regular rhythm, 150/min
- Normal axis (R and S waves equal in lead I)
- QRS complex duration 120 ms (upper limit of normal)
- The second R peak (R^1) is taller than the R peak

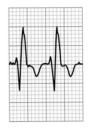

R^1 taller than R peak in lead V$_1$

Broad complex tachycardia of uncertain origin

Note
- Regular rhythm, 195/min
- Right axis deviation (suggests a supraventricular tachycardia with bundle branch block)
- Very broad QRS complexes, with duration 200 ms (the primary evidence for ventricular tachycardia)
- QRS complexes in lead V$_1$ point upwards, while complexes in V$_6$ point downwards: no concordance (suggests a supraventricular tachycardia)
- The second R peak (R^1) is greater than the first R peak in lead V$_1$ (suggests a supraventricular tachycardia)

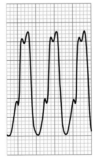

Broad complexes

137

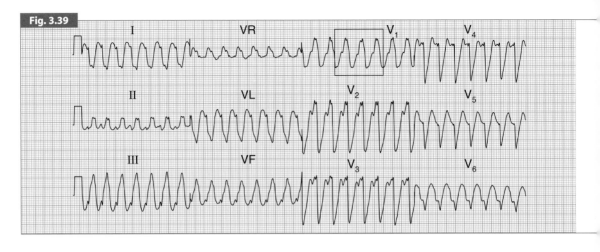

Fig. 3.39

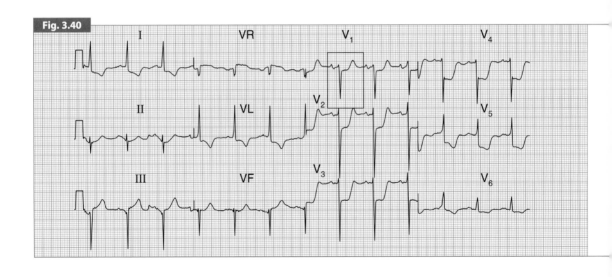

Fig. 3.40

Broad complex tachycardia: ?ventricular, ?supraventricular
Note
- Regular rhythm, 180/min
- Right axis deviation
- Very broad complexes, with QRS complex duration 200 ms
- R and R¹ peaks are variable
- No concordance

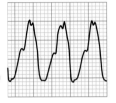

Variable R and R¹ peaks in lead V_1

Often only a comparison of the patient's ECGs taken in sinus rhythm and when the tachycardia is present will establish the nature of the tachycardia. In the case of any patient with a tachycardia it is essential to look through the old notes, to see if any ECGs have been recorded previously. The ECG in Figure 3.39 shows the broad complex tachycardia of a patient who was in pain and was hypotensive. He was cardioverted, and Figure 3.40 shows the post-cardioversion record. The QRS complexes are narrow, so the arrhythmia must have been VT.

Post-cardioversion: sinus rhythm with normal conduction
Note
- Same patient as in Figure 3.39
- Sinus rhythm
- Axis now shows left deviation
- Narrow QRS complexes
- Widespread ST segment depression, indicating ischaemia
- The narrow QRS complexes, with a change of axis, show that the original rhythm (shown in Fig. 3.39) must have been ventricular

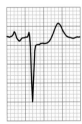

Narrow QRS complexes in lead V_1

139

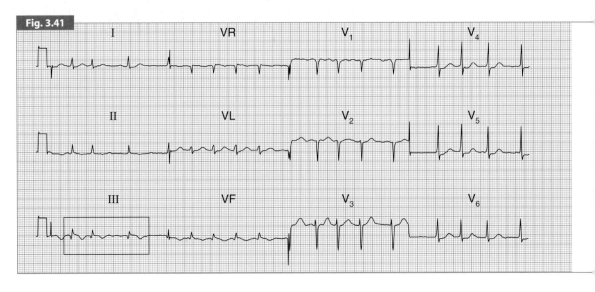

Fig. 3.41

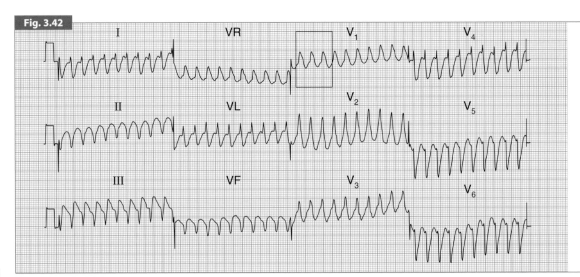

Fig. 3.42

Atrial fibrillation and inferior infarction

Note
- Irregular, narrow complex rhythm
- Irregular baseline indicates atrial fibrillation
- Normal axis
- Small Q waves in leads III and VF with inverted T waves, suggesting inferior infarction
- Slight ST segment depression in leads V_4–V_5 suggests ischaemia

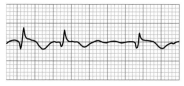

Small Q waves and inverted T waves in lead III

Figure 3.41 shows the ECG from a patient admitted to hospital with an inferior myocardial infarction, initially with atrial fibrillation. The patient then developed a broad complex tachycardia (Fig. 3.42). In the context of an acute infarction this would almost certainly be VT. A comparison of Figures 3.41 and 3.42 shows the development of a different, indeterminate, axis and of RBBB. The change of axis is a strong pointer to a ventricular origin of the rhythm.

Ventricular tachycardia (VT) and inferior infarction

Note
- Same patient as in Figure 3.41
- Broad complex tachycardia
- Indeterminate axis
- Right bundle branch block (RBBB) pattern, but in lead V_1, R peak greater than R^1 peak (not very clearly defined)
- No concordance
- With acute myocardial infarction, this will be VT

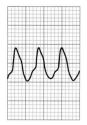

RBBB pattern in lead V_1

141

Fig. 3.43

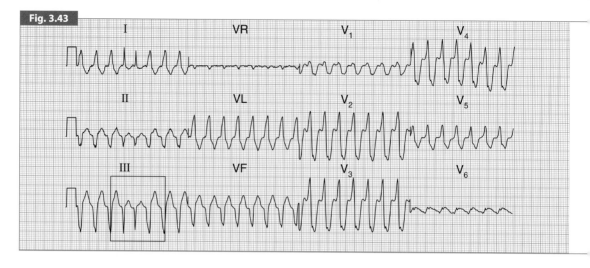

FUSION BEATS AND CAPTURE BEATS

If an early beat can be found with a narrow QRS complex, it can be assumed that a wide complex tachycardia is ventricular in origin. The narrow early beat demonstrates that the bundle branches will conduct supraventricular beats normally, even at high heart rates.

A 'fusion beat' is said to occur when the ventricles are activated simultaneously by a supraventricular and a ventricular impulse, so that a QRS complex with an intermediate pattern is seen (Fig. 3.43). The appearance of fusion beats is variable.

A 'capture beat' occurs when the ventricles are activated by an impulse of supraventricular origin during a run of VT (also shown in Fig. 3.43), and so capture beats have a QRS complex like those seen in a supraventricular rhythm. Figure 3.44 shows another example of a capture beat, indicating that the broad complex tachycardia is VT.

Ventricular tachycardia

Note

- Broad complex tachycardia, 180/min
- Left axis deviation
- Probable right bundle branch block (RBBB) pattern, with R peak greater than R^1 in lead V_1
- Two narrow complexes in leads I–III – the first is probably a 'fusion' beat and the second a 'capture' beat

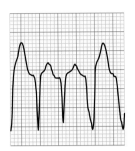

Fusion and capture beats in lead III

Fig. 3.44

Ventricular tachycardia

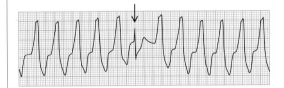

Note

- A single early beat with a narrow QRS complex (arrowed) interrupts a broad complex tachycardia
- A single 'capture' beat must have a supraventricular origin, and by inference the broad complexes must have a ventricular origin

DIFFERENTIATION OF BROAD COMPLEX TACHYCARDIAS

Box 3.5 summarizes some distinguishing features of broad complex tachycardias.

SPECIAL FORMS OF VENTRICULAR TACHYCARDIA IN PATIENTS WITH SYMPTOMS

RIGHT VENTRICULAR OUTFLOW TRACT TACHYCARDIA (RVOT-VT)

This is usually an exercise-induced tachycardia, which originates in the right ventricular outflow tract. It is recognizable because the broad complex tachycardia shows a combination of right axis deviation and left bundle branch block (Fig. 3.45). RVOT-VT can be treated by ablation.

TORSADE DE POINTES

Ventricular tachycardia (VT) is called 'monomorphic' when all the QRS complexes have the same appearance, and 'polymorphic' when they vary. A 'twisting' or 'writhing' polymorphic VT is called 'torsade de pointes'. This is often seen in patients whose ECG in sinus rhythm shows a long QT interval (see pp. 48 and 76). Figures 3.46 and 3.47 show the ECGs from a patient with a long QT interval when in sinus rhythm, who developed torsade de pointes VT. This pattern immediately raises the possibility of drug toxicity, and in this case the cause was a tricyclic antidepressant (see p. 77).

Figure 3.48 shows another example of torsade de pointes VT, in this case due to a Class I antiarrhythmic drug.

Possible causes of torsade de pointes VT due to drugs are listed in Box 3.6.

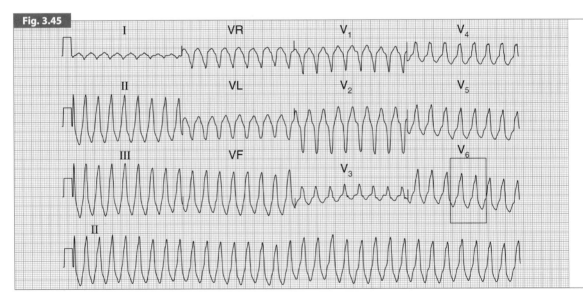

Fig. 3.45

Box 3.5 Differentiation of broad complex tachycardias

- Broad complex tachycardias in patients with acute myocardial infarction are likely to be ventricular
- Compare with record taken in sinus rhythm – change of axis suggests a ventricular rhythm
- Left axis deviation, especially with right bundle branch block, is usually ventricular
- Identify P waves (independent P waves may be seen in ventricular tachycardia)
- QRS complex width: if > 160 ms, usually ventricular
- QRS complex regularity: if very irregular, probably atrial fibrillation with conduction defect
- Concordance: ventricular tachycardia is likely if the QRS complexes are predominantly upward, or predominantly downward, in all the chest leads
- With right bundle branch block pattern, ventricular origin is likely if:
  — there is left axis deviation
  — the primary R wave is taller than the secondary R wave (R^1) in lead V_1
- With left bundle branch block pattern, ventricular origin is likely if there is a QS wave (i.e. no R wave) in lead V_6
- Capture beats: narrow complex following short R–R interval (i.e. an early narrow beat interrupting a broad complex tachycardia) suggests that the basic rhythm is ventricular
- Fusion beats: an intermediate QRS complex pattern arises when the ventricles are activated simultaneously by a supraventricular and a ventricular impulse

Right ventricular outflow tract ventricular tachycardia

Note

- Broad complex tachycardia
- Right axis deviation
- Left bundle branch block (LBBB) pattern

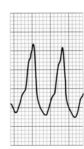

Broad QRS complexes and LBBB pattern in lead V_6

Fig. 3.46

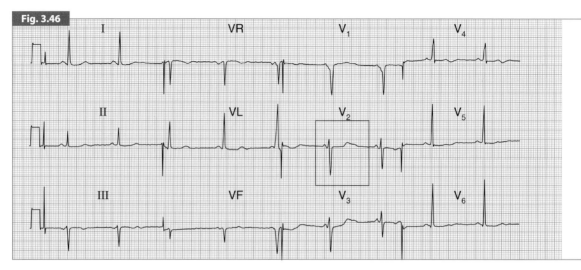

Fig. 3.47

Torsade de pointes ventricular tachycardia

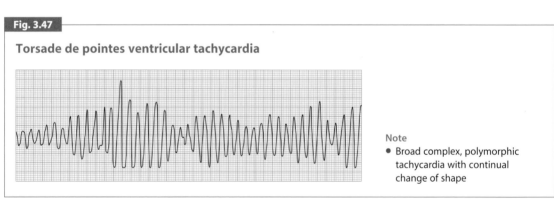

Note
- Broad complex, polymorphic tachycardia with continual change of shape

Box 3.6 Drugs causing torsade de pointes ventricular tachycardia

- Class I antiarrhythmic drugs
- Amiodarone
- Sotalol
- Tricyclic antidepressants
- Many other drugs

Long QT syndrome: drug toxicity

Note
- Sinus rhythm
- Third complex in lead VL is probably a 'fusion' beat
- QT interval difficult to measure because of U waves, but probably about 540 ms

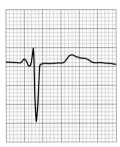

Long QT interval in lead V_2

Fig. 3.48

Torsade de pointes ventricular tachycardia

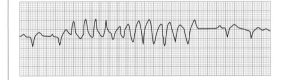

Note
- Two sinus beats are followed by ventricular tachycardia
- The complexes initially point upwards, but then become inverted; the QRS complex rate is variable

---

TACHYCARDIAS ASSOCIATED WITH THE WOLFF–PARKINSON–WHITE SYNDROME

In patients with an accessory pathway due to the Wolff–Parkinson–White (WPW) syndrome, the more common (orthodromic) re-entry tachycardia involves narrow QRS complexes, and thus it resembles a supraventricular tachycardia, unless bundle branch block is present (see p. 69).

If conduction within the re-entry circuit is antidromic, the ECG will show a wide QRS complex which can look remarkably like VT.

In a patient with the WPW syndrome and a tachycardia with a cause other than a re-entry circuit, such

147

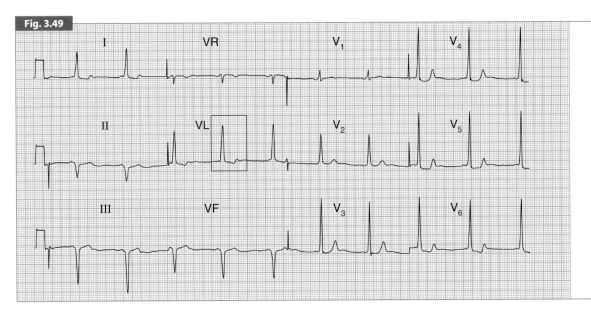

Fig. 3.49

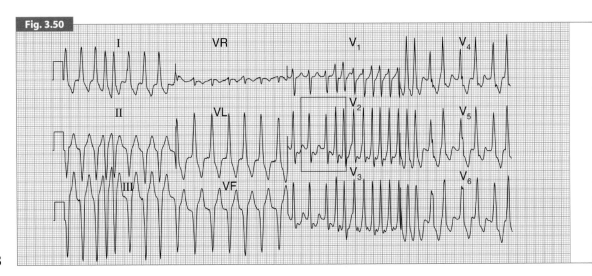

Fig. 3.50

The Wolff–Parkinson–White syndrome, type A

Note

- Sinus rhythm
- Short PR interval
- Left axis deviation
- Prominent delta wave
- Dominant R waves in lead V_1, indicating type A WPW

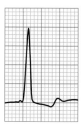

Short PR interval and delta wave in lead VL

as atrial fibrillation, the accessory pathway may have no significant role, and is then described as a 'bystander'. The tachycardia will have broad complexes, even when conduction in both the His bundle and the accessory pathway is anterograde. With atrial fibrillation, the complexes will be polymorphic (variable-shape) and very irregular. This is extremely dangerous, because if the fast-conducting accessory pathway becomes involved and conducts depolarization associated with atrial flutter or fibrillation to the ventricles, the result can be ventricular fibrillation (Figs 3.49 and 3.50).

The Wolff–Parkinson–White syndrome with atrial fibrillation

Note

- Same patient as in Figure 3.49
- Irregular broad complex tachycardia
- Rate up to 300/min
- Delta waves still apparent
- Marked irregularity suggests atrial fibrillation

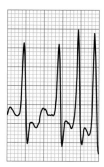

Delta waves in lead V_2

149

MANAGEMENT OF ARRHYTHMIAS

WHAT TO DO WHEN AN ARRHYTHMIA IS SUSPECTED

1. Consider possible underlying diagnoses.
2. Simple investigations:
   — haemoglobin (sinus tachycardia)
   — thyroid function (sinus tachycardia, bradycardia or atrial fibrillation)
   — chest X-ray (for heart size and to exclude the possibility of mild heart failure).
3. Ambulatory ECG: 24-h recording if symptoms are frequent, or event recording when symptoms are infrequent.
4. Echocardiography, to aid diagnosis when any sort of structural heart disease seems possible (e.g. valve disease with atrial fibrillation, or cardiomyopathy with syncope).
5. Tilt testing, when neurocardiogenic syncope or orthostatic hypotension (rather than an arrhythmia) is suspected.

PRECIPITATION OF ARRHYTHMIAS

Arrhythmias are sometimes precipitated by exercise (Fig. 3.51), and if the patient's history suggests that this is so, then treadmill testing may be helpful. Attempts to provoke an arrhythmia by exercise should, however, only be made when full resuscitation facilities are available.

If the patient complains of syncopal attacks, particularly on movement of the head, it is worth pressing the carotid sinus in the neck to see if the patient has carotid sinus hypersensitivity. Complete SA node inhibition may be induced, sometimes with unpleasant effects (Fig. 3.52).

WHAT TO DO WHEN AN ARRHYTHMIA IS RECORDED

- Does the arrhythmia need treating as an emergency?
  — If there are unpleasant symptoms, or evidence of haemodynamic disturbance – yes.
  — If the patient is asymptomatic – probably not, unless haemodynamic problems seem likely.
- Does the arrhythmia have an obvious cause? Some possible causes of palpitations are listed in Box 3.7.
- Consider the principles of arrhythmia management:
  — Any arrhythmia causing significant symptoms or a haemodynamic disturbance must be treated immediately.
  — All antiarrhythmic drugs should be considered cardiac depressants, and they are potentially pro-arrhythmic. The use of multiple agents should be avoided.
  — Electrical treatment (cardioversion for tachycardias, pacing for bradycardias) should be used in preference to drug therapy when there is marked haemodynamic impairment.

Fig. 3.51

Exercise-induced ventricular tachycardia

Rest

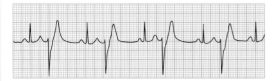

Exercise

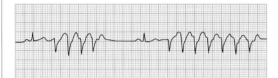

Note
● At rest (upper trace) the ECG shows frequent ventricular extrasystoles
● During exercise (lower trace), ventricular tachycardia occurs

Fig. 3.52

Carotid sinus hypersensitivity

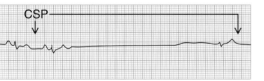

Note
● Carotid sinus pressure causes cessation of all cardiac activity, due to excessive vagal influence

CAROTID SINUS PRESSURE IN THE MANAGEMENT OF TACHYCARDIAS

The first step in the management of any tachycardia is to try carotid sinus pressure (CSP).

In sinus rhythm, CSP will cause transient slowing of the heart rate. This may be useful in identifying the true origin of the rhythm when there is doubt (Fig. 3.53).

In atrial flutter, AV conduction is blocked so the ventricular rate falls. The atrial activity becomes obvious, which helps to identify the rhythm (Fig. 3.54). CSP seldom converts atrial flutter to sinus rhythm.

In atrial tachycardia and junctional tachycardia, CSP may restore sinus rhythm (Fig. 3.55).

In atrial fibrillation and ventricular tachycardia, CSP has no effect.

EXTRASYSTOLES

- Supraventricular: no treatment. If the patient has symptoms, explanation and reassurance. Advise to discontinue smoking and avoid coffee and alcohol.
- Ventricular: usually no treatment, though treatment may be considered:
  — when ventricular extrasystoles are so frequent that cardiac output is impaired
  — when there is a frequent R on T phenomenon
  — when the patient complains of an irregular heartbeat but reassurance and an explanation prove ineffective.
- Three ventricular extrasystoles together (a 'salvo') should be treated as a ventricular tachycardia.

Box 3.7 Causes of palpitations associated with various cardiac rhythms

Extrasystoles
- Normal heart
- Any cardiac disease
- Anaemia

Sinus tachycardia
- Normal heart
- Anxiety
- Anaemia
- Acute blood loss
- Thyrotoxicosis
- Pregnancy
- Lung disease
- CO_2 retention
- Pulmonary embolus
- Phaeochromocytoma
- Sympathomimetic drugs, including inhalers and caffeine

Atrial fibrillation
- Rheumatic heart disease
- Thyrotoxicosis
- Ischaemic heart disease
- Cardiomyopathy
- Alcoholism
- Apparently normal heart with 'lone atrial fibrillation'

Supraventricular tachycardia
- Pre-excitation syndromes
- Apparently normal heart

Ventricular tachycardia
- Acute myocardial infarction
- Ischaemic heart disease
- Cardiomyopathy (hypertrophic or dilated)
- Long QT syndrome
- Myocarditis
- Drugs
- Apparently normal heart: idiopathic

Fig. 3.53

CSP and sinus rhythm

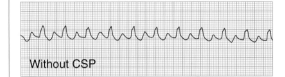

Without CSP

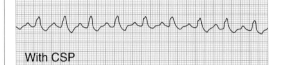

With CSP

Note
- Upper trace shows a broad complex tachycardia
- It is not obvious whether the deflection before the QRS complex represents a T wave, or a T wave followed by a P wave
- Lower trace shows that with CSP the rate falls, and P waves become obvious

Fig. 3.54

CSP in atrial flutter

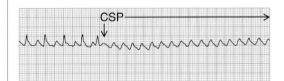

Note
- CSP increases the block at the AV node
- Ventricular activity is completely suppressed
- Flutter waves are obvious

Fig. 3.55

CSP in junctional tachycardia

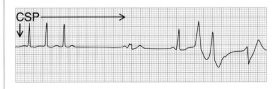

Note
- CSP reverts junctional tachycardia to sinus rhythm, but in this case multifocal ventricular extrasystoles occurred

153

SINUS TACHYCARDIA

Remember that sinus tachycardia always has a cause (see Box 3.7), and it is the cause that should be treated.

ATRIAL TACHYCARDIA

Remember that this may be due to digoxin toxicity. Treat as for AVNRT (see below).

ATRIOVENTRICULAR NODAL RE-ENTRY TACHYCARDIA (AVNRT, JUNCTIONAL TACHYCARDIA)

Try, in this order:

1. Carotid sinus massage.
2. Adenosine 3 mg i.v. bolus, followed if necessary after 2 min by a further 6 mg adenosine and, if necessary after a further 2 min, by a further 12 mg adenosine. Unwanted but transient effects include asthma, flushing, chest tightness and dizziness.
3. Verapamil 2.5–5 mg i.v. or atenolol 2.5 mg i.v., repeated at 5 min intervals to a total of 10 mg. Note: These drugs should not be administered together, and verapamil should not be given to patients receiving a beta-blocker.
4. DC shock.

ATRIAL FIBRILLATION AND FLUTTER

A choice has to be made between rate control and conversion of atrial fibrillation to sinus rhythm. It should be remembered that long-term success following conversion is very unlikely in patients who:

- have had atrial fibrillation for more than a year
- have cardiac enlargement
- have any form of structural abnormality in the heart.

If a patient has a ventricular rate of > 150/min and chest pain or other evidence of poor perfusion, immediate cardioversion should be attempted. In an emergency, immediate heparin treatment provides adequate prophylaxis against embolism. Cardioversion can be attempted with amiodarone i.v. or flecainide i.v., but electrical cardioversion (100 J–200 J–360 J) is more reliable.

Patients who are not haemodynamically impaired, and who have been in atrial fibrillation for more than 24 h, should be treated with warfarin before cardioversion is attempted. Effective anticoagulation (INR > 2.0) is needed for at least 1 month before the procedure.

For rate control, use one of:

- i.v. amiodarone
- i.v. verapamil
- i.v. beta-blocker
- i.v. digoxin 250 μg by slow injection, repeated at 30 min intervals to a total of 1 mg,

and remember the need for anticoagulants.

PREVENTION OF PAROXYSMAL ATRIAL FIBRILLATION

Atrial fibrillation is called 'paroxysmal' if there are attacks that revert spontaneously; 'persistent' if the rhythm is continuous but cardioversion has not been attempted; and 'permanent' if cardioversion has failed.

Digoxin will probably not prevent attacks of atrial fibrillation, but the prophylactic use of some drugs may prevent attacks for months, or possibly years:

- sotalol
- flecainide (avoid in patients with coronary disease)
- amiodarone.

These drugs can be used after DC cardioversion, but at best only about 40% of patients will still be in sinus rhythm after a year.

Electrophysiological ablation is an option (see below) and in very resistant cases, electrical ablation of the AV node can be used to cause complete heart block, and a permanent pacemaker inserted.

VENTRICULAR TACHYCARDIA

Ventricular tachycardia (VT) can be treated with one of:

- Lidocaine 100 mg i.v., repeated twice at 5 min intervals, followed by a lidocaine infusion at 2–3 mg/min.
- Amiodarone 300 mg i.v. over 30 min then 900 mg over 24 h, followed by 200 mg t.d.s. by mouth for 1 week, 200 mg b.d. for 1 week and 200 mg daily thereafter.
- Atenolol 2.5 mg i.v., repeated at 5 min intervals to 10 mg.
- Flecainide 50–100 mg i.v., or 100 mg b.d. by mouth – but avoid in patients with coronary disease.
- Magnesium 8 mmol i.v. over 15 min, followed by 64 mmol over 24 h.

Note: When amiodarone is given i.v. a deep vein must be used. Overdose prolongs the QT interval and can cause VT. Long-term treatment may cause skin pigmentation, photosensitive rashes, abnormalities of thyroid or liver function, drug deposits in the cornea, or, occasionally, pulmonary fibrosis.

Second-line drugs for VT include disopyramide and mexiletine. Recurrent episodes, which cannot be controlled by drugs, are treated with an implanted defibrillator.

Patients with congenital long QT syndromes and paroxysmal VT are treated in the first instance with beta-blockers, or with an implanted defibrillator.

THE WOLFF–PARKINSON–WHITE SYNDROME

Adenosine, digoxin, verapamil and lidocaine may increase conduction through the accessory pathway and block it in the AV node. This can be extremely dangerous if atrial fibrillation occurs, because it may lead to ventricular fibrillation. These drugs should therefore not be used for the treatment of pre-excitation tachycardias.

Drugs that slow conduction in the accessory pathway are:

- atenolol
- flecainide
- amiodarone.

These drugs can be used for prophylaxis against paroxysmal arrhythmias, but the definitive treatment is electrical ablation of the accessory pathway.

ELECTROPHYSIOLOGY AND CATHETER ABLATION

When drug treatment fails, or for some reason is inappropriate, some tachyarrhythmias can be treated by the electrical ablation of an abnormal conducting pathway. This has first to be identified by electrophysiology.

THE ENDOCARDIAL ECG

Electrical mapping catheters introduced via a transvenous route into the heart can be used to measure the pattern of electrical activation in the heart. Usually catheters are placed in the right atrium, the right ventricle, across the tricuspid valve (close to the His bundle), and in the coronary sinus (to measure the pattern of left ventricular depolarization). Figure 3.56 shows an X-ray taken during a fairly typical investigation, with exploring electrodes in different cardiac chambers. More sophisticated mapping catheters, including looped catheters and balloon catheters, may be employed in more complex cases.

Fig. 3.56

Still fluoroscopic image of transvenous catheters during electrophysiology

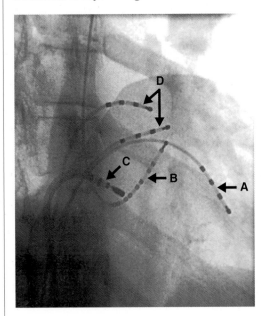

Note
- Catheters have multiple electrodes (dark bands) to enable mapping of the propagation of endocardial electrical activity
- Catheters shown are: right ventricular (A), coronary sinus (B), His bundle (C) and atrial (D)

CATHETER ABLATION

If an abnormal conduction pathway, e.g. in the Wolff–Parkinson–White syndrome, can be located (mapped) and permanently interrupted, a paroxysmal re-entry tachycardia can be prevented and the patient can be cured without the need for further drug therapy. This used to be done surgically, but now abnormal re-entry pathways are ablated (cauterized) by burning with radiofrequency energy applied through an intracardiac catheter. Ablation can also be used to destroy a focus of enhanced automaticity or triggered activity that is the cause of an arrhythmia.

The endocardial ECG is used to identify both the mechanism of an arrhythmia and the optimal position for the administration of a catheter-mediated radiofrequency ablation burn. The resting pattern of the cardiac electrical activity, as well as the pattern of activity in response to atrial or ventricular pacing and attempted pharmacological stimulation of the arrhythmia, may be recorded during electrophysiological studies. Real-time analysis of the endocardial ECG allows the precise assessment of the relative timing of atrial and ventricular depolarization in different anatomical positions within the heart. This in turn provides information on the propagation of depolarization. Abnormal sources or routes of depolarization can then be mapped, and a position identified for radiofrequency ablation.

An example of the use of the endocardial ECG in catheter ablation is shown in Figure 3.57. It is important to recognize that the paper speed used in electrophysiology is usually greater than that used for 12-lead ECGs, and so the scale of the trace differs. Figure 3.57 shows continuous traces from surface ECG leads I and V_1. Intracardiac electrograms are recorded at the proximal (CS-prox) and distal (CS-dist) poles of a multipolar catheter placed in the coronary sinus (CS) (Fig. 3.56). The coronary sinus runs in the groove of the left atrioventricular sulcus, so both atrial (A) and ventricular (V) electrograms are recorded. The atrial electrograms from the coronary sinus arise from atrial tissue close to the AV junction. These areas depolarize late in atrial systole, so coincide with the end of the P wave seen in the surface ECG leads. The final electrogram shown in Figure 3.57 was recorded from the tip of the mapping/ablation catheter (MAP). This single-tip catheter is used as a mapping electrode, to probe for the optimal site for ablation, and is also used to deliver the radiofrequency ablation burn once this position is found.

The first three beats recorded in Figure 3.57 show sinus rhythm, conducted with pre-excitation via a left-sided accessory pathway – with a negative delta wave in lead I, positive delta wave in lead V_1, and closely spaced atrial (A) and ventricular (V) electrograms recorded by the CS catheter. On applying radiofrequency energy for ablation (RF on), there was an almost immediate loss of pre-excitation, with the disappearance of delta waves in the ECG leads in the following beats. The interval between atrial and ventricular electrograms within each beat increased at the CS catheter, indicating normal conduction via the AV node and no conduction via the accessory pathway. The PR interval also increased, from less than 120 ms in the first three beats to 180 ms, following successful radiofrequency ablation of the accessory pathway.

ARRHYTHMIAS AMENABLE TO ABLATION

ATRIAL FLUTTER

Typical atrial flutter results from a re-entry circuit within the atria. This can be abolished by ablating an area known as the right atrial isthmus, which prevents re-entry from occurring (Fig. 3.58).

ATRIAL FIBRILLATION

There is increasing evidence that in a high proportion of patients atrial fibrillation is initiated either by enhanced atrial automaticity or by triggered activity arising in the vicinity of the pulmonary veins, probably in atrial tissue extending into the pulmonary venous ostia and in the atrial area immediately outside the venous ostia. Ablation (Fig. 3.59) can isolate the atrial tissue within the pulmonary veins from the rest of the atrium, and hence can suppress the initiation of paroxysmal atrial fibrillation and also reduce relapse after the cardioversion of permanent atrial fibrillation.

The ablation treatment of atrial fibrillation is more difficult than that of atrial flutter, because the left atrium has to be entered through the inter-atrial septum, involving trans-septal puncture through the foramen ovale, and more burns are needed. It is usually initially performed with a wide-area circumferential ablation (WACA, denoted by red dots in Fig. 3.59). Further segmental ablation, guided by pacing from a coronary sinus electrode, may be required to eliminate persisting areas of conduction until the pulmonary veins are electrically silent. At present this technique is usually regarded as a second-line option, limited to patients with symptoms refractory to conventional medical therapy, although its wider application is the subject of ongoing study.

AV NODE ABLATION

Patients with atrial-driven tachyarrhythmias, especially atrial fibrillation (whether paroxysmal or permanent), which cannot be controlled by pharmacological means, may undergo catheter ablation of the AV node. This leads to complete AV block, and bradycardia is prevented by the implantation of a permanent pacemaker ('ablate and pace').

PATHWAY ABLATION

Atrioventricular re-entry tachycardias, such as in the Wolff–Parkinson–White syndrome, can be treated by ablation of the accessory pathway, as described above. This prevents re-entry and eliminates pre-excitation and episodes of supraventricular tachycardia. The ablation of pathways close to the AV node, including those involved in atrioventricular nodal re-entry tachycardia (AVNRT), can be attempted. The aim of ablation is to modify the slow pathway, and so prevent AVNRT, without damaging the fast pathway, which would lead to AV block and necessitate a permanent pacemaker.

Fig. 3.57

Endocardial ECG: ablation of left-sided accessory pathway

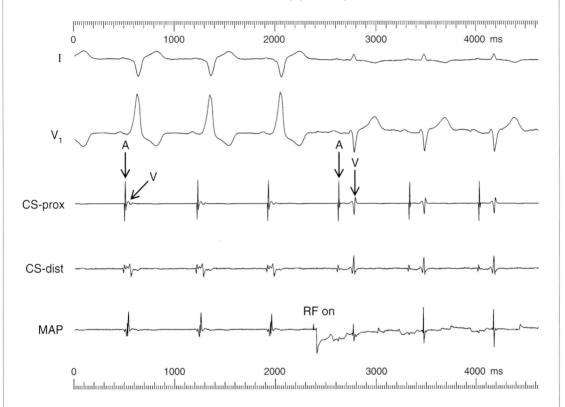

Note
- Increased paper speed compared to 12-lead ECG
- Delta wave in first three beats: positive in lead V_1, negative in lead I, PR interval < 120 ms
- Atrial (A) and ventricular (V) depolarization are almost superimposed before ablation, indicating conduction via an accessory pathway
- After ablation (RF on): delta wave in leads I and V_1 is lost; increased PR interval (180 ms); increased separation of atrial and ventricular depolarization recorded in the coronary sinus. These changes indicate AV nodal conduction

Fig. 3.58

Typical atrial flutter ablation

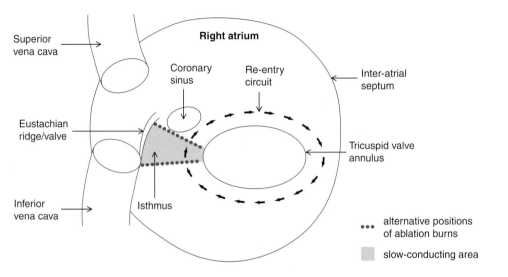

Note
- Arrhythmia occurs due to a clockwise or counter-clockwise re-entry circuit around the tricuspid valve annulus
- The re-entry circuit requires conduction through a narrow 'isthmus' of slow-conducting tissue (shaded grey) between the tricuspid valve annulus, the inferior vena cava, the coronary sinus and the Eustachian ridge/valve
- Radiofrequency ablation of this isthmus interrupts and prevents re-entry

Fig. 3.59

Ablation for atrial fibrillation

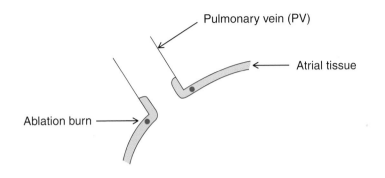

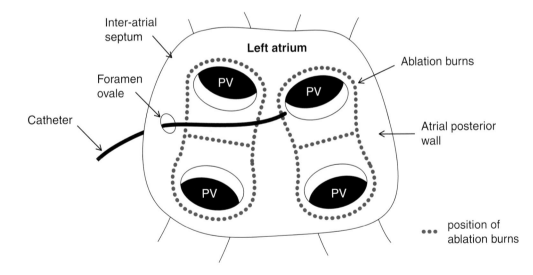

Note
- Anatomy of pulmonary venous drainage is variable. Most commonly four veins drain into the posterior left atrium

VENTRICULAR TACHYCARDIA

Some forms of ventricular tachycardia (VT) are amenable to catheter radiofrequency ablation treatment. These include right ventricular outflow tract VT, where triggered activity is the cause, and also VT in some patients with surgically corrected congenital heart disease, if a simple ventricular re-entry circuit can be demonstrated. Ischaemic VT is not usually amenable to electrophysiological ablation, because often there are multiple potential foci of increased automaticity and potential re-entry circuits, due to areas of myocardial scarring. More sophisticated ventricular mapping tools are becoming available which potentially enable ablation treatment even for ischaemic VT.

INDICATIONS FOR ELECTROPHYSIOLOGY

The indications for electrophysiology, and the associated hazards, are summarized in Box 3.8.

CARDIAC ARREST

The ECG in Figure 3.60 was being recorded from a patient with an acute inferior myocardial infarction when he collapsed due to VF. Patients who survive ventricular fibrillation should be considered for the insertion of an implanted cardioverter defibrillator (ICD) (see below).

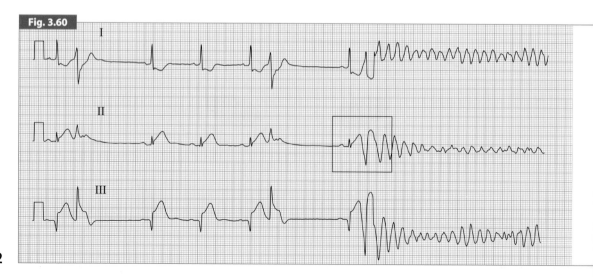

Fig. 3.60

Box 3.8 **Indications and complications of electrophysiology**

Indications
- Atrioventricular re-entry tachycardias, including the Wolff–Parkinson–White syndrome
- Atrial fibrillation or atrial flutter, either paroxysmal or permanent, where the symptoms are refractory to conventional therapy or where medical therapy is contraindicated or poorly tolerated
- AV node ablation for paroxysmal or permanent atrial arrhythmias (especially atrial fibrillation) refractory to rate control with conventional medical therapy
- AV node slow pathway modification for symptomatic/medication-refractory AVNRT
- Ventricular tachycardias outside the context of ischaemic heart disease, including those associated with congenital heart disease and right ventricular outflow tract ventricular tachycardia
- Non-sustained ventricular tachycardia, as part of preparation for an ICD device (see indications for ICD devices): a ventricular tachycardia stimulation study
- Symptomatic or frequent ventricular extrasystoles, especially if associated with a significant cardiomyopathy

Complications
- Peri-procedural stroke or TIA (transient ischaemic attack) (1%)
- Groin haematoma (7%)
- Pericardial tamponade (1%)
- Arteriovenous fistula (< 1%)
- Higher degree AV block (with pathways close to the AV node)
- Pulmonary vein stenosis (1%) (pulmonary vein isolation only)
- Repeated procedures (complex studies may require repeat procedures)

Ventricular fibrillation
Note
- Leads I, II and III, continuous records
- Initially sinus rhythm, with occasional ventricular extrasystoles
- R on T ventricular extrasystole followed by ventricular fibrillation

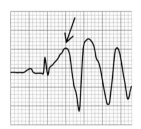

R on T phenomenon in lead II

MANAGEMENT OF CARDIAC ARREST

The treatment of an individual patient will depend on the particular arrhythmia involved. Remember, confirm cardiac arrest by checking (ABC):

- Airway
- Breathing
- Circulation.

The immediate actions are:

- Begin cardiopulmonary resuscitation (CPR). Ventilation and chest compression should be given in a ratio of 2 breaths to every 30 compressions.
- Defibrillate in cases of ventricular fibrillation and pulseless ventricular tachycardia as soon as possible.
- Intubate as soon as possible.
- Gain or verify IV access.

SHOCKABLE RHYTHMS – VENTRICULAR FIBRILLATION (VF) OR PULSELESS VENTRICULAR TACHYCARDIA (VT)

Actions:

1. Precordial thump (especially useful in VT).
2. Defibrillate at 200 J.
3. 2 min of CPR.
4. If unsuccessful, defibrillate at 360 J.
5. If unsuccessful, give adrenaline (epinephrine) 1 mg i.v.
6. Defibrillate at 360 J.
7. 2 min of CPR.
8. If VF/pulseless VT persists, give amiodarone 300 mg i.v.
9. Give further shocks after 2-min periods of CPR.
10. Give adrenaline (epinephrine) 1 mg i.v. immediately before alternate shocks.
11. For refractory VF, give magnesium sulfate 2 g i.v. bolus (8 mmol).

The ECG in Figure 3.61 shows a successful defibrillation.

NON-SHOCKABLE RHYTHMS – ASYSTOLE AND PULSELESS ELECTRICAL ACTIVITY (PEA)

The term 'PEA' has replaced 'electromechanical dissociation' (EMD) because some pulseless patients have weak myocardial contractions, although insufficient to generate a cardiac output. In cases of PEA, think about the underlying causes.
Actions:

- Precordial thump.
- CPR 30:2 (30 chest compressions followed by 2 ventilations).
- If it is unclear whether the rhythm is 'fine ventricular fibrillation' or asystole, treat as VF until three defibrillations have not changed the apparent rhythm.
- Adrenaline (epinephrine) 1 mg i.v.
- CPR 30:2 for 2 min.
- Atropine 3 mg i.v.
- If unsuccessful, continue adrenaline (epinephrine) 1 mg after alternate 2-min cycles of CPR.

Fig. 3.61

DC conversion of ventricular fibrillation

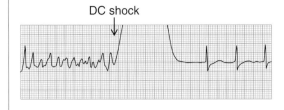

DC shock

Note
- Ventricular fibrillation is abolished by DC shock
- A supraventricular rhythm (probably sinus in origin) immediately takes control of the heart

CAUSES OF CARDIAC ARREST

With any case of cardiac arrest, consider the possibility of a reversible cause (all of which begin with **H** or **T**):

- Hypoxia.
- Hypovolaemia.
- Hyperkalaemia, hypokalaemia, hypocalcaemia, acidosis, hypoglycaemia.
- Hypothermia.
- Tension pneumothorax.
- Tamponade.
- Toxic substances, or therapeutic substances in overdose.
- Thromboembolic or mechanical obstruction (e.g. pulmonary embolus).

Following resuscitation, check:

- Arterial blood gases – if the pH is < 7.1 or if arrest is associated with tricyclic overdose, give bicarbonate 50 mmol.
- Electrolytes.
- ECG.
- Chest X-ray – principally to exclude a pneumothorax caused by the resuscitation.

IMPLANTED CARDIOVERTER DEFIBRILLATOR (ICD) DEVICES

These devices are designed for patients who have survived ventricular fibrillation or are at increased risk of ventricular arrhythmia or sudden cardiac death. They have the following functions:

- pacemaker
- defibrillator
- control of ventricular tachycardia.

PACEMAKER FUNCTION

ICD devices have the same functions as a conventional pacemaker (see Ch. 4). They can be single or dual chamber, or biventricular (CRTD). In patients who do not require the pacing function, the ICD will usually be a single-chamber system, programmed as a backup VVI. The device will then be in continuous sensing mode.

Fig. 3.62

Chest X-ray showing single chamber ICD

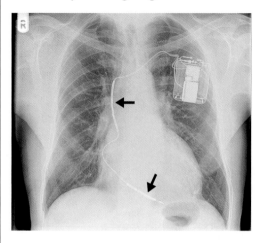

Note
- Single right ventricular lead, with thicker areas indicating the poles of the shocking coils (arrowed)

Fig. 3.63

ICD cardioversion of ventricular fibrillation

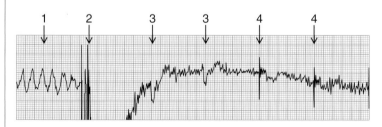

Note
- Ventricular fibrillation (1) followed by ICD-mediated cardioversion (2)
- Intrinsic QRS complexes (3)
- Paced ventricular responses (4)

DEFIBRILLATOR FUNCTION

The chest X-ray appearances of ICD devices are similar to those of conventional pacemakers. However, devices with a defibrillating function are bigger, incorporating more battery power for the delivery of shocks. In addition, the right ventricular lead contains the two poles of the shocking coil and so is thicker than a conventional lead (Fig. 3.62).

In addition to the normal sensing functions of a pacemaker, an ICD can sense high rates of ventricular activity. If a predetermined ventricular rate is exceeded, an electrical shock discharges between the two poles of the defibrillator coil in the ventricular lead, with the aim of cardioverting a life-threatening ventricular arrhythmia (Fig. 3.63). If the ventricular rate does not fall below the threshold following one shock, then further shocks may be delivered.

ANTI-TACHYCARDIA PACING

The device may also attempt to control ventricular tachycardia by 'overdrive pacing'. If ventricular activity is detected within a certain range (usually significantly above normal cardiac rates but below the threshold set for defibrillation), the ICD will attempt to pace the ventricle at a high rate before reducing the rate of pacing. Ventricular capture with rapid pacing can sometimes terminate ventricular tachycardia. If anti-tachycardia pacing in this way is unsuccessful after a set number of attempts, the ICD will then usually default to defibrillation.

Box 3.9 **Indications for ICD insertion**

'Primary' prevention
- Previous myocardial infarction (MI) (> 4 weeks previously) and ejection fraction < 35% (but symptoms no worse than NYHA Class III) *and* non-sustained ventricular tachycardia (VT) on Holter monitoring *and* inducible VT on electrophysiology
- Previous MI (> 4 weeks previously) and ejection fraction < 30% (but symptoms no worse than NYHA Class III) *and* QRS complexes < 120 ms
- Familial risk of sudden cardiac death including hypertrophic cardiomyopathy, long QT syndrome, Brugada syndrome, or ARVD (arrhythmogenic right ventricular dysplasia)
- Surgical repair of congenital heart disease

Secondary prevention
- Survived cardiac arrest due to ventricular fibrillation or VT
- Spontaneous sustained VT causing syncope or haemodynamic compromise
- Sustained VT and ejection fraction < 35% (but symptoms no worse that NYHA Class III)

INDICATIONS FOR ICD DEVICES

These are summarized in Box 3.9.

ECG APPEARANCE

ECGs from patients with ICDs are the same as those from patients with conventional pacemakers, except when a ventricular arrhythmia is detected.

ABNORMAL ICD FUNCTION

Either the pacing function or the defibrillator function of an ICD device may fail. The defibrillator function may either fail appropriately to initiate ventricular arrhythmia therapy, or may deliver inappropriate shocks. This will require specialist input and analysis. In the event of inappropriate repeated shock delivery, an ICD can be inactivated in a monitored patient by the application of a magnet.

ICDs should always be interrogated shortly after shock delivery, even if this was appropriate, to check device function and battery life. The presence of pacemakers or ICDs in no way precludes external defibrillation, provided that the paddles are not applied directly over the device.

The ECG when the patient has a bradycardia

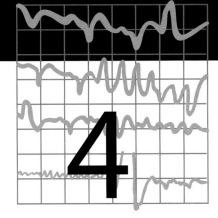

4

Mechanism of bradycardias	**169**
Sinoatrial disease – the 'sick sinus syndrome'	171
Atrial fibrillation and flutter	176
Atrioventricular block	179
Management of bradycardias	**187**
Temporary pacing in patients with acute myocardial infarction	187
Permanent pacing	187
Right ventricular pacemakers (VVI)	189
Right atrial pacemakers (AAI)	197
Dual-chamber pacemakers (DDD)	199
Abnormal pacemaker function	202
Indications for pacemaker insertion	206

MECHANISM OF BRADYCARDIAS

Patients are seldom aware that their heart rate is slow, but they can certainly be aware of the effects of a bradycardia. Marked sinus bradycardia is characteristic of athletic training, but it is also a contributory cause of the symptom of fainting in vasovagal attacks, the reduced cardiac output and syncope associated with heart block, and hypotension and heart failure in patients with an inferior myocardial infarction. A slow heart rate can also be a major contributor to angina. An ECG is therefore an essential part of the investigation of any patient with a slow pulse rate, and indeed of any patient with dizziness, syncope or breathlessness.

The causes of sinus bradycardia have been discussed in Chapter 1 (see Box 1.2, p. 5). Escape rhythms have been discussed in Chapter 2 (p. 82). They are usually asymptomatic, but symptoms occur when the automaticity that generates the escape rhythm is inadequate to maintain a cardiac output. A bradycardia may cause the symptom of syncope; some of the possible underlying causes are listed in Box 4.1.

Box 4.1 Conditions associated with syncope

Atrial fibrillation with slow ventricular rate
- Rheumatic heart disease
- Ischaemic heart disease
- Cardiomyopathies
- Drugs:
  - digoxin
  - beta-blockers
  - verapamil
  - amiodarone

'Sick sinus' disease
- Congenital
- Familial
- Idiopathic
- Ischaemic heart disease
- Rheumatic heart disease

- Cardiomyopathy
- Amyloidosis
- Collagen diseases
- Myocarditis
- Drugs, e.g. lithium

Second or third degree block
- Idiopathic (fibrosis)
- Congenital
- Ischaemia
- Aortic valve calcification
- Surgery or trauma
- Tumours in the His bundle
- Drugs:
  - digoxin
  - beta-blockers

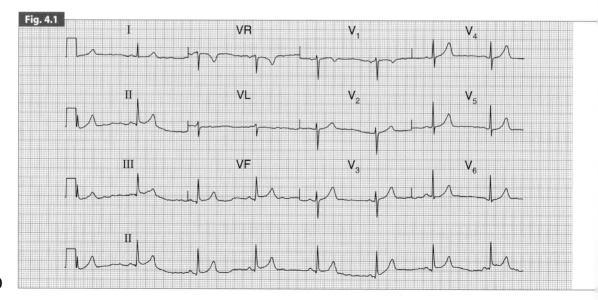

Fig. 4.1

SINOATRIAL DISEASE – THE 'SICK SINUS SYNDROME'

Disordered SA node function can be familial or congenital and can occur in ischaemic, rheumatic, hypertensive or infiltrative cardiac disease. It is, however, frequently idiopathic. Abnormal function of the SA node may be associated with failure of the conduction system. Many patients with sinoatrial disease are asymptomatic, but all the symptoms associated with bradycardias – dizziness, syncope and the symptoms of heart failure – can occur. Atrial and junctional tachycardias often occur together with sinus node dysfunction, when the patient may present with palpitations.

The abnormal rhythms seen in the sick sinus syndrome are listed in Box 4.2.

The ECGs in Figures 4.1 and 4.2 are from a young man who had a normal ECG with a slow sinus rate when asymptomatic, but intermittently became extremely dizzy when he developed a profound sinus bradycardia.

The ECG in Figure 4.3 shows an ambulatory record from a young woman who complained of short-lived attacks of dizziness. When she had these, the ECG showed sinus pauses.

Figure 4.4 shows the other variety of sinus pause – sinus arrest.

The ECG in Figure 4.5 shows an example of a 'silent atrium', when the heart rhythm depends on the irregular depolarization of a focus in the AV node.

The combination of sick sinus syndrome and episodes of tachycardia is sometimes called the 'bradycardia–tachycardia syndrome' and Figure 4.6 shows the rhythm of a patient with this syndrome. This patient was asymptomatic at times, when his ECG showed a 'silent atrium' with a slow and irregular junctional (AV nodal) escape rhythm, but he complained of palpitations when he had an AV nodal tachycardia.

Sinus bradycardia

Note
- Sinus rhythm
- Rate 45/min, ECG otherwise normal

Box 4.2 **Cardiac rhythms in the sick sinus syndrome**

- Unexplained or inappropriate sinus bradycardia
- Sudden changes in sinus rate
- Sinus pauses (sinoatrial arrest or exit block)
- Atrial standstill ('silent atrium')
- Atrioventricular junctional escape rhythms
- Atrial tachycardia alternating with junctional escape (bradycardia–tachycardia syndrome)
- Junctional tachycardia alternating with junctional escape
- Atrial fibrillation with a slow ventricular response
- Prolonged pauses after premature atrial beats

Fig. 4.2

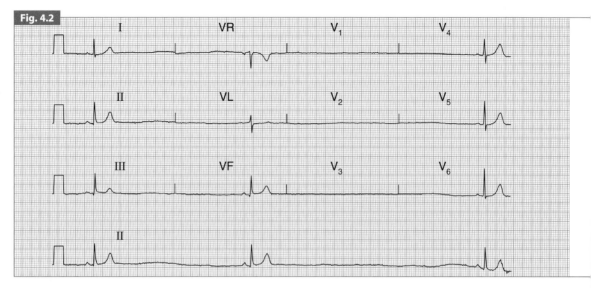

Fig. 4.3

Sinus pauses

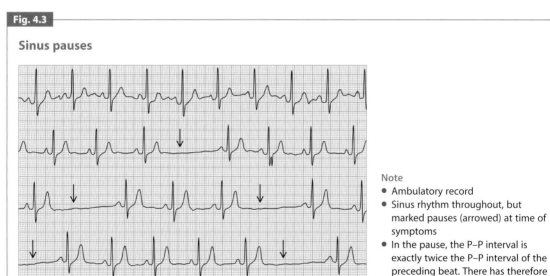

Note
- Ambulatory record
- Sinus rhythm throughout, but marked pauses (arrowed) at time of symptoms
- In the pause, the P–P interval is exactly twice the P–P interval of the preceding beat. There has therefore been 'exit block' from the SA node

Sick sinus syndrome: sinus bradycardia

Note
- Same patient as in Figure 4.1
- Sinus rhythm
- Rate down to 12/min at times
- No complexes recorded in leads V_1–V_3

Fig. 4.4

Sinus arrest

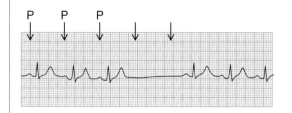

Note
- Sinus rhythm
- After three beats there is a 'sinus pause' with no P wave
- Arrows mark where the next two P waves should have been
- Sinus rhythm is then restored, but the cycle has been reset

Fig. 4.5

Sick sinus syndrome: silent atrium

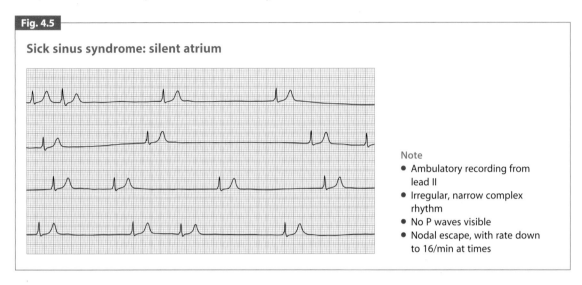

Note
- Ambulatory recording from lead II
- Irregular, narrow complex rhythm
- No P waves visible
- Nodal escape, with rate down to 16/min at times

Fig. 4.7

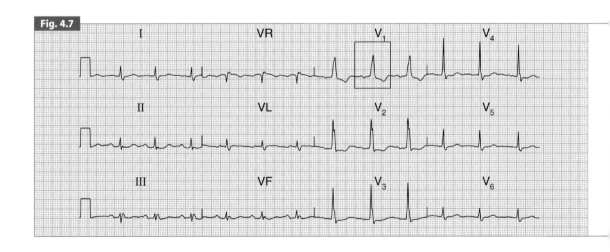

Fig. 4.6

Sick sinus syndrome: bradycardia–tachycardia syndrome

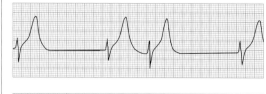

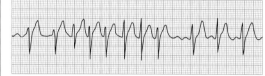

Note
- Upper trace: a silent atrium with irregular junctional escape beats
- Lower trace: junctional tachycardia is followed by a period of sinus rhythm

First degree block and right bundle branch block

Note
- Sinus rhythm
- PR interval 220 ms (first degree block)
- Right bundle branch block (RBBB)

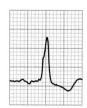

Long PR interval and RBBB pattern in lead V_1

Figure 4.7 shows the ECG from a patient who, when asymptomatic, showed first degree block and right bundle branch block. He complained of fainting attacks, and an ambulatory recording showed that this was due to sinus arrest with a very slow AV nodal escape rhythm, giving a ventricular rate of 15/min (Fig. 4.8, p. 177). This is an example of the combination of conduction system disease and sick sinus syndrome.

Possible causes of sick sinus syndrome are listed in Box 4.3.

Fig. 4.8

Sinus arrest and atrioventricular nodal escape

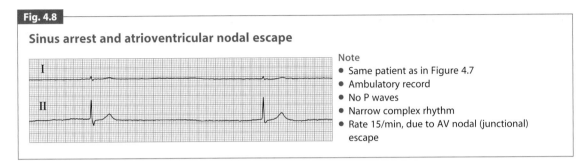

Note
- Same patient as in Figure 4.7
- Ambulatory record
- No P waves
- Narrow complex rhythm
- Rate 15/min, due to AV nodal (junctional) escape

ATRIAL FIBRILLATION AND FLUTTER

A slow ventricular rate can accompany atrial flutter or atrial fibrillation because of slow conduction through the AV node and His bundle systems (Figs 4.9 and 4.10). This may be the result of treatment with drugs that delay AV nodal conduction, such as digoxin, beta-blockers or verapamil, but can occur because of conducting tissue disease.

Complete block associated with atrial fibrillation is recognized from the regular and wide QRS complexes which originate in the ventricular muscle (Fig. 4.11).

Fig. 4.9

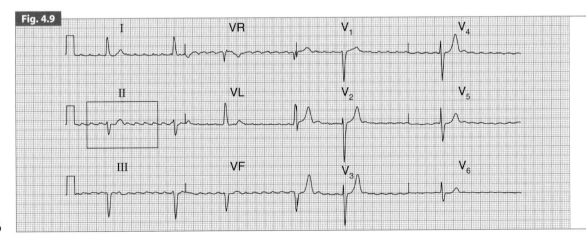

Box 4.3 **Causes of the sick sinus syndrome**

Familial
- Isolated
- With atrioventricular conduction disturbance
- With QT interval prolongation
- Congenital

Acquired
- Idiopathic
- Coronary disease
- Rheumatic disease
- Cardiomyopathy
- Neuromuscular disease:
  — Friedreich's ataxia
  — peroneal muscular atrophy
  — Charcot–Marie–Tooth disease

- Infiltration:
  — amyloidosis
  — haemochromatosis
- Collagen diseases:
  — rheumatoid
  — scleroderma
  — systemic lupus erythematosus
- Myocarditis:
  — viral
  — diphtheria
- Drugs:
  — lithium
  — aerosol propellants

Atrial flutter with variable block

Note
- Irregular bradycardia
- Flutter waves at 300/min obvious in all leads
- Ventricular rate varies, range 30–55/min
- QRS complex duration slightly prolonged (128 ms), indicating partial right bundle branch block
- There is not complete block, as shown by the irregular QRS complexes

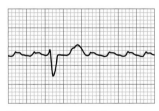

Flutter waves in lead II

Fig. 4.10

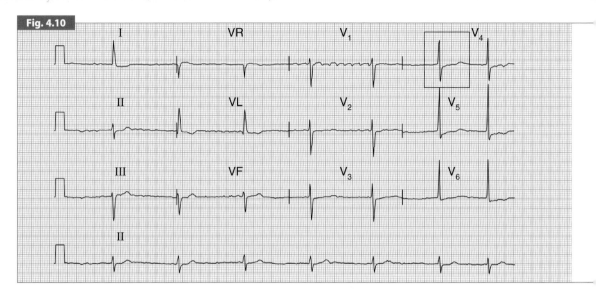

Fig. 4.11

Atrial fibrillation and complete block

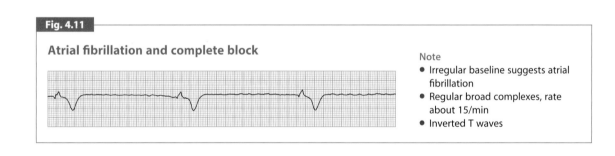

Note
- Irregular baseline suggests atrial fibrillation
- Regular broad complexes, rate about 15/min
- Inverted T waves

Atrial fibrillation

Note

- Irregular rhythm, rate 43/min
- Flutter-like waves in lead V_1 but these are not constant
- Left axis deviation
- QRS complexes otherwise normal
- Prolonged QT intervals of 530 ms: ?hypokalaemia

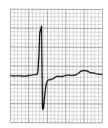

Prolonged QT interval in lead V_4

ATRIOVENTRICULAR BLOCK

Symptoms are not caused by first degree block, second degree block of the Wenckebach or Mobitz type 2 varieties, left anterior hemiblock or the bundle branch blocks.

Second degree block of the 2:1 or 3:1 type will cause dizziness and breathlessness if the ventricular rate is slow enough (Fig. 4.12). Young people tolerate slow hearts better than old people do.

Complete (third degree) block characteristically involves a slow rate, but this may be fast enough to cause only tiredness or the symptoms of heart failure.

Figure 4.13 shows the ECG of a 60-year-old man who, despite a heart rate of 40/min, had few complaints.

If the ventricular rate is very slow the patient may lose consciousness in a 'Stokes–Adams' attack, which can cause a seizure and sometimes death. The ECG in Figure 4.14 is from a patient who was asymptomatic while his ECG showed sinus rhythm with first degree block and right bundle branch block, but who then had a Stokes–Adams attack with the onset of complete block (Fig. 4.15).

The possible causes of heart block are summarized in Box 4.4.

Fig. 4.12

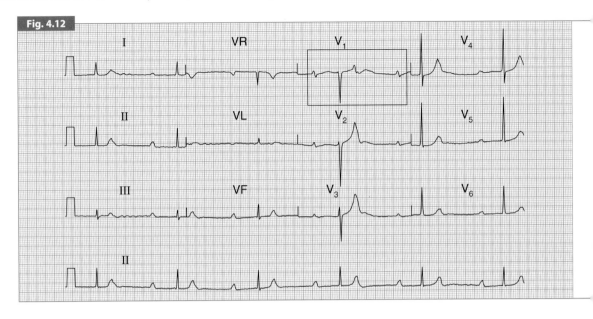

Fig. 4.13

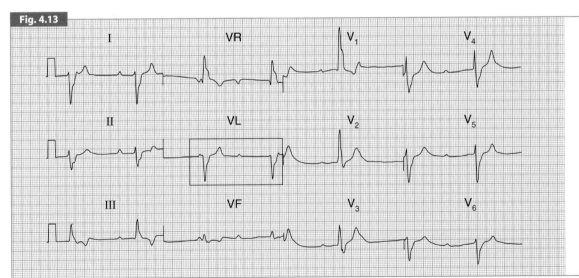

Second degree block (2:1)

Note

- Sinus rhythm
- Second degree block, 2:1 type
- Ventricular rate 33/min
- Long PR interval in the conducted beats (not characteristic of second degree block)
- Normal QRS complexes and T waves

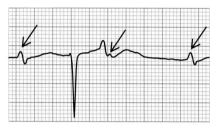

P waves in lead V₁

Complete heart block

Note

- Sinus rate 70/min
- Regular ventricular rate, 40/min
- No relationship between P waves and QRS complexes
- Wide QRS complexes
- Right bundle branch block pattern

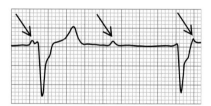

P waves in lead VL

181

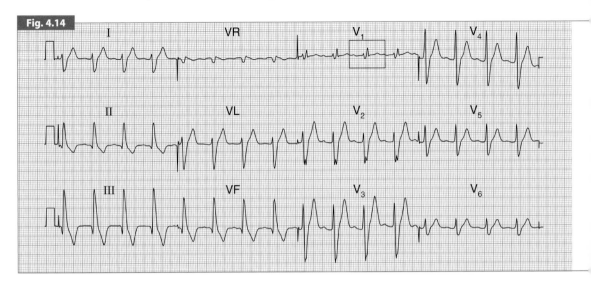

Fig. 4.14

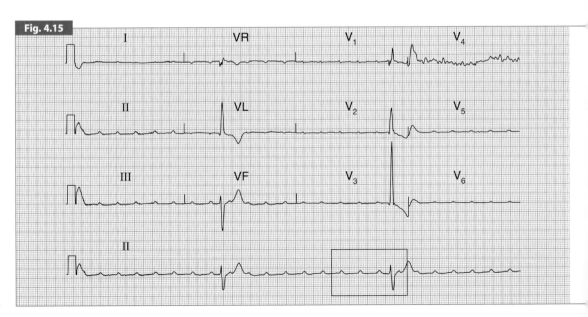

Fig. 4.15

First degree block and right bundle branch block

Note

- Sinus rhythm
- PR interval 240 ms
- Right axis deviation
- Right bundle branch block (RBBB)

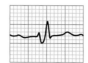

Long PR interval and RBBB pattern in lead V_1

Complete block and Stokes–Adams attack

Note

- Same patient as in Figure 4.14
- Sinus rate 140/min
- Ventricular rate 15/min
- No relationship between P waves and QRS complexes
- Because of the slow ventricular rate, no QRS complexes were recorded in leads I–III or V_1–V_3, although the rhythm strip shows a complex in lead II

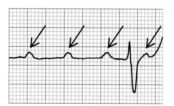

P waves

Box 4.4 **Causes of heart block**

First and second degree block	Complete block
• Normal variant	• Idiopathic (conduction tissue fibrosis)
• Increased vagal tone	• Congenital
• Athletes	• Ischaemic disease
• Sick sinus syndrome	• Associated with aortic valve calcification
• Acute carditis	• Cardiac surgery and trauma
• Ischaemic disease	• Digoxin intoxication
• Hypokalaemia	• Bundle interruption by tumours, parasites, abscesses,
• Lyme disease (*Borrelia burgdorferi*)	granulomas, injury
• Digoxin	
• Beta-blockers	
• Calcium-channel blockers	

THE ENDOCARDIAL ECG IN ATRIOVENTRICULAR BLOCK

The ordinary surface ECG provides all the information necessary for the identification of heart block, but the spread of excitation through the heart can be seen more accurately from an intracardiac recording.

The endocardial ECG used during electrophysiological studies simultaneously displays depolarizations recorded from several catheters, passed percutaneously via a vein in to the heart. Each catheter has multiple electrodes (see Fig. 3.56), which show the timing of depolarization through the heart (Fig. 4.16). The components of the wave of depolarization are best illustrated from recordings taken by the His catheter. The 'A' wave of atrial depolarization (the P wave of the surface ECG) is normally followed by the sharp deflection of the 'H' spike, caused by the depolarization of the His bundle. The AH interval is 55–120 ms in normal subjects, with most of this period being due to delay within the AV node. The 'V' wave normally follows, representing ventricular depolarization (the QRS complex of the surface ECG). The HV interval (normal range 33–35 ms) measures the time taken for depolarization to spread from the His bundle to the first part of the interventricular septum.

Figure 4.17 shows an endocardial ECG from a patient with first degree heart block, in this case due to prolongation of the AH interval.

A His bundle electrogram also demonstrates the site of second degree block. In the case of 2:1 block, this is usually in the His bundle rather than the AV node. Therefore a normal H (or His) spike will be seen, but in the nonconducted beats the H spike will not be followed by a V wave (Figs 4.18 and 4.19).

Fig. 4.16

Normal His bundle electrogram

P QRS T P QRS T P QRS
A H V A H V
40 ms intervals

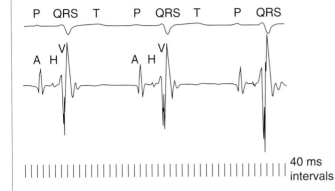

Note
- Upper trace shows the usual ECG recorded from the body surface
- The P waves, QRS complexes and T waves are broad and flat because the record was made with a faster paper speed than normal
- The lower trace shows the intracardiac recording. The A and V waves correspond to the P waves and QRS complexes, but have a totally different appearance
- His bundle depolarization is shown as a small spike labelled 'H'

Fig. 4.17

His electrogram: first degree block

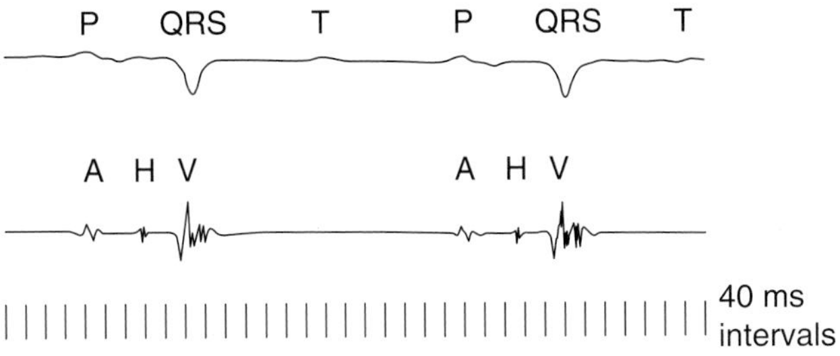

P QRS T P QRS T
A H V A H V
40 ms intervals

Note
- Upper record shows surface ECG
- PR interval 200 ms
- Lower record shows His electrogram
- AH interval is prolonged (150 ms), but the HV interval is normal (70 ms)

Fig. 4.18

Second degree block (2:1)

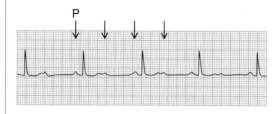

Note
- The conducted beats have a normal PR interval
- Alternate P waves are not followed by a QRS complex

Fig. 4.19

His electrogram: second degree block

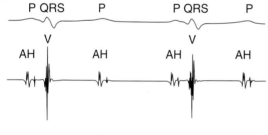

40 ms intervals

Note
- Upper trace shows the surface ECG
- As in the case of other His electrograms, the paper speed is fast – so the P–QRS–T complexes are flattened and spread out
- Lower trace shows first a normal A wave, H spike and V wave, but then an A wave and an H spike with no V wave
- The sequence is then repeated

MANAGEMENT OF BRADYCARDIAS

Bradycardias must be treated if they are associated with hypotension, poor peripheral perfusion, or escape arrhythmias. Any bradycardia can be treated with:

- Atropine 600 µg i.v., repeated at 5 min intervals to a total 1.8 mg. Note: Overdose causes tachycardia, hallucinations and urinary retention.
- Isoprenaline 1–4 µg/min. Note: Overdose causes ventricular arrhythmias which are difficult to treat. An isoprenaline infusion should only be used while preparations are being made for pacing.

TEMPORARY PACING IN PATIENTS WITH ACUTE MYOCARDIAL INFARCTION

Bradyarrhythmias associated with an acute myocardial infarction, especially those with an inferior infarction, usually resolve spontaneously, without the need for pacemaker insertion. However, temporary pacing is indicated with:

- complete block with ventricular rate < 50/min and hypotension
- any persistent bradycardia needing an isoprenaline infusion.

Prolonged monitoring is needed in the case of the deterioration of patients with the following conditions, with a view to temporary pacing if necessary:

- any complete block
- second degree block with heart rate < 50/min
- bundle branch block plus first degree block
- bifascicular block plus first degree block
- evidence of increasing block
- bradycardia with escape rhythms
- drug-induced tachyarrhythmias.

PERMANENT PACING

Pacemakers and other cardiac devices are increasingly prevalent, especially in elderly patients. Although usually implanted and monitored by specialists, these devices are frequently encountered in a broad range of clinical contexts. The different types of pacemaker can be characterized by the number of cardiac chambers involved. Patients often carry a card indicating the type of device implanted, but this can also be determined by its characteristic appearance on a plain chest X-ray. A chest X-ray is, therefore, a necessary part of any pacemaker assessment, and so this chapter includes a series of X-rays. It is essential that the type of device be determined before the ECG can be interpreted.

All pacemakers perform two fundamental functions: pacing and sensing. Most ECG findings in both normal and abnormal pacemaker function can be explained in terms of pacing and sensing functions.

PACING

An electrical pulse is generated between an electrical pole at the tip of the pacing lead and either a second pole more proximally within the pacing lead (bipolar lead) or the pacemaker box itself (unipolar lead). This causes depolarization of the surrounding myocardium, the propagation of an action potential from this focus and the contraction of the paced cardiac chamber. This process is repeated at a basal rate determined when the pacemaker is programmed, although it can be suppressed as a result of device sensing (see below).

SENSING

The pacemaker continuously monitors electrical activity in the vicinity of the tip of the pacing lead.

If intrinsic cardiac depolarization is sensed in a single-chamber pacemaker, the pacemaker will inhibit pacing for a predetermined period. This prevents simultaneous pacing in the presence of spontaneous cardiac activity.

In dual-chamber pacemakers, sensing depolarization can either inhibit pacing in the same chamber or trigger pacing in a different chamber. For example, if an intrinsic ventricular beat is sensed, ventricular pacing will be inhibited for a period. If atrial depolarization is sensed, ventricular pacing will be triggered after a programmed PR interval, but only if no ventricular activity has been sensed. Thus ventricular pacing can track atrial activity in the presence of AV block, leading to appropriate coordination of atrial and ventricular systole.

PACEMAKER NOMENCLATURE

The pacing mode of most pacemaker systems can be described using the NBG Code (NASPE/BPEG Generic, developed by the North American Society of Pacing and Electrophysiology Mode Code Committee and the British Pacing and Electrophysiology Group).

The letters of the NBG Code signify the following:

A = right atrium
V = right ventricle
D = dual
0 = none
I = inhibited

In the code:

- the first letter describes the chamber(s) paced (A, V or D)
- the second letter describes the chamber(s) sensed (A, V, D or 0)
- the third letter describes the response to a sensed event (I, D or 0)
- a fourth letter (R) is used when the rate modulation is programmable.

The most commonly used types of pacemaker are listed in Table 4.1.

Table 4.1 **Types of pacemaker**

Nomenclature	Chamber(s) with impanted electrode	Device function
Single chamber		
VVI	RV	RV sensed, RV paced Sensed event inhibits pacemaker
AAI	RA	RA sensed, RA paced Sensed event inhibits pacemaker
VVI/ICD	RV	RV sensed, RV paced Sensed event inhibits pacemaker In case of ventricular fibrillation, ICD defibrillates
Dual chamber		
DDD	RA RV	RA and RV sensed, RA and RV paced Sensed event inhibits pacemaker
DDD/ICD	RA – pacing lead RV – pacing and shocking lead	RA and RV sensed, RA and RV paced Sensed event inhibits pacemaker In case of ventricular fibrillation, ICD defibrillates

ICD, implantable cardioverter defibrillator; LA, left atrium; LV, left ventricle; RA, Right atrium; RV, right ventricle.

RIGHT VENTRICULAR PACEMAKERS (VVI)

One of the most common types of pacemaker, these have a single lead implanted in the right ventricle, usually at the apex (Fig. 4.20). The lead senses electrical activity in the right ventricle and, if no spontaneous cardiac activity is sensed, paces the ventricle after a predetermined interval. Note that unipolar and bipolar pacing leads cannot easily be differentiated on a routine chest X-ray. The indications for VVI pacing are listed in Box 4.5.

Box 4.5 **Indications for VVI pacing**

- Atrial fibrillation with a slow ventricular rate or pauses
- Sinoatrial disease (bradycardia–tachycardia syndrome), in which patients have atrial-driven tachyarrhythmias (such as fast atrial fibrillation) but periods of relative bradycardia that prevent pharmacological rate control
- 'Backup' pacemaker, in patients with occasional pauses due to sinus node disease or atrioventricular block but a predominantly spontaneous cardiac rhythm
- In the very elderly, in whom more sophisticated devices are unlikely to improve function

189

Fig. 4.20

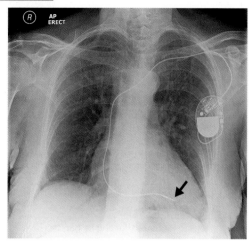

Chest X-ray showing right ventricular pacemaker

Note
- Pacemaker unit positioned in a subcutaneous pocket beneath the left shoulder
- Pacing lead passing via the subclavian vein, with the lead tip in the conventional right ventricular apical position (arrowed)

Fig. 4.21

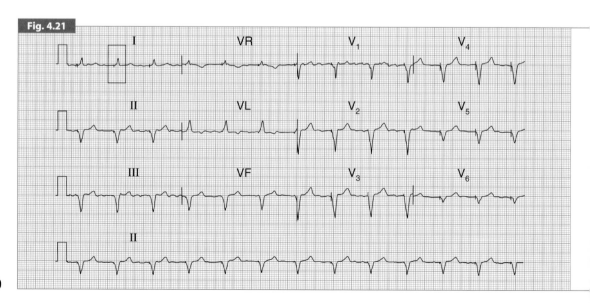

ECG APPEARANCE

With bipolar right ventricular pacing, the ECG is characterized by a pacing spike followed by a broad QRS complex of left bundle branch block morphology, because cardiac depolarization originates from the lead tip in the right ventricle (Fig. 4.21). The pacing spikes vary in size and morphology in different ECG leads and in different patients, and may not be visible in all leads.

With unipolar pacing, in which the electrical circuit is between the lead tip and the pacemaker box, the pacing spike is very large compared to that associated with bipolar pacing, in which the poles are close together (Fig. 4.22).

If the pacemaker senses spontaneous cardiac activity, pacing will be suppressed for a predetermined time interval. The ECG will then show intermittent pacing, with varying amounts of paced ventricular rhythm and underlying ventricular rhythm (Figs 4.23 and 4.24).

The ECGs of patients with pacemakers programmed to provide a backup function for occasional slow rhythms may show no paced beats at all, if the intrinsic cardiac rate exceeds the programmed pacing rate.

VVI bipolar pacing

Note

- Pacing spike followed by a paced ventricular beat with a broad complex. Because the paced complex originates from the right ventricle, its morphology is similar to that seen in left bundle branch block
- The size of the pacing spike varies in different ECG leads, and it may not be visible
- The unchanging morphology of the QRS complex in the rhythm strip confirms continuous right ventricular pacing
- Underlying atrial fibrillation (best seen in lead V_1)

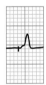

Pacing spike followed by broad QRS complex

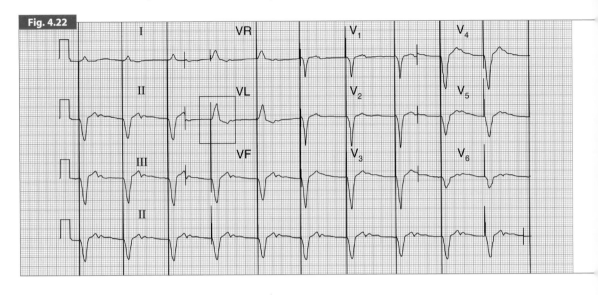

Fig. 4.22

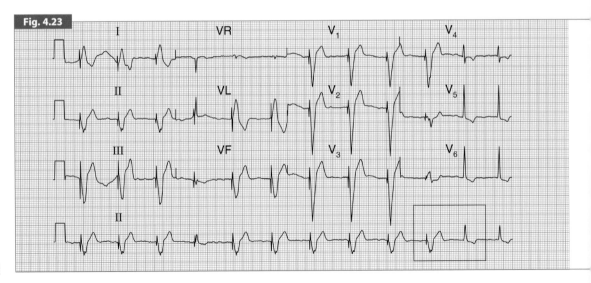

Fig. 4.23

VVI unipolar pacing

Note

- Pacing spikes much larger than with bipolar pacing

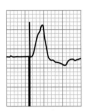

Large ventricular pacing spike

Intermittent VVI pacing

Note

- Ventricular pacing
- Underlying rhythm can be seen to be atrial fibrillation
- Final two beats with narrow complexes are not paced – the intrinsic heart rate exceeds that of the pacemaker

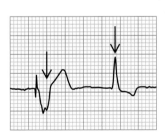

First beat paced, second beat unpaced

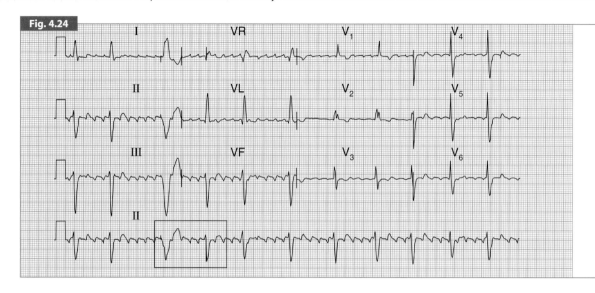

Fig. 4.24

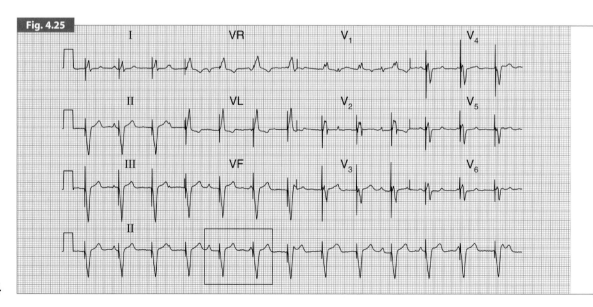

Fig. 4.25

Atrial flutter with intermittent VVI pacing
Note
- Underlying atrial flutter with variable block
- After the second beat the subsequent pause exceeds the trigger rate for the pacemaker, and the third beat shows ventricular pacing
- All other QRS complexes are intrinsic (i.e. not paced), indicating normal ventricular sensing
- Vertical lines where the lead changes (e.g. from VL to V_2) must not be confused with pacing spikes

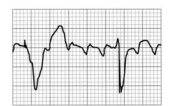

First beat paced, second beat intrinsic

VVI pacing: complete block
Note
- Ventricular pacing
- P waves can be seen, unrelated to ventricular beats
- Therefore the underlying rhythm is complete heart block

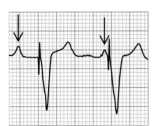

Complete block (P waves arrowed)

The underlying atrial rhythm can be determined from the ECG, and may be important for clinical decisions, such as anticoagulation. There may be sinus rhythm, atrial fibrillation, atrial flutter (Fig. 4.24) or complete block (Fig. 4.25).

EXTRA FUNCTIONS

Rate response modulation (VVIR) allows an increase in the pacing rate to a preset higher level in the presence of increased activity, as detected from movement. This facilitates some increase in the heart rate with exercise.

195

Fig. 4.26

Chest X-ray showing right atrial pacemaker

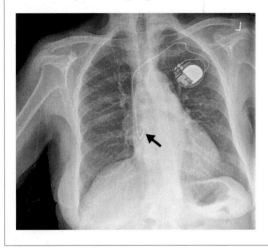

Note
- Pacemaker unit positioned in the left prepectoral position
- The single atrial lead passes via the subclavian vein to the right atrial appendage (arrowed)

Fig. 4.27

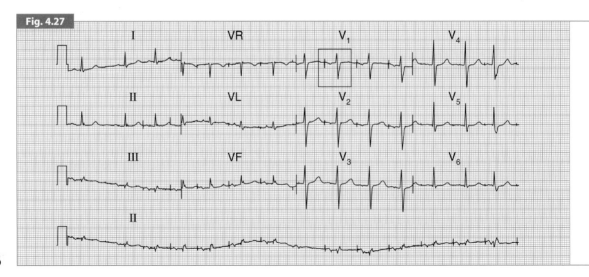

RIGHT ATRIAL PACEMAKERS (AAI)

This is a rarely used mode of pacing, with a single lead implanted in the right atrium, usually in the atrial appendage (Fig. 4.26). This type of pacing senses spontaneous activity in the right atrium, and paces if the sinus node rate falls below a predetermined level.

The indications for AAI pacing are summarized in Box 4.6.

Box 4.6 Indications for AAI pacing

- Sinus node disease with no evidence of atrioventricular node disease
- Young patients with symptomatic sinus pauses

AAI pacing
Note
- Pacing spike precedes each P wave
- The subsequent QRS complex is normal, with no evidence of AV block

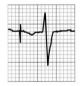

Atrial pacing spike, normal PR interval, normal QRS complex

ECG APPEARANCE

With atrial pacing the ECG is characterized by a pacing spike followed by a paced P wave. The PR interval and QRS complex are usually normal, indicating no AV node disease (Fig. 4.27).

With intermittent pacing, if the pacemaker senses spontaneous atrial activity, atrial pacing will be suppressed for a predetermined period. Atrial pacemakers are usually implanted to provide backup during fairly rare sinus pauses. Therefore, most of the time a normal ECG, with no paced beats, would be expected.

EXTRA FUNCTIONS

Rate response modulation (AAIR) allows an increase in pacing rate to a preset higher level in the presence of increased activity, as detected from movement. This allows some increase in the heart rate with exercise.

The 'rate drop response' allows the pacemaker to respond to sudden decreases in atrial rate by pacing at a higher rate, and is designed to try to prevent loss of consciousness during episodes of neurocardiogenic syncope.

Fig. 4.28

Chest X-ray showing dual chamber pacemaker

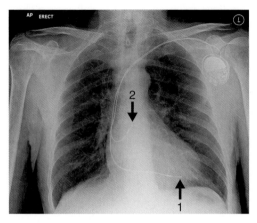

Note
- Pacemaker unit in the left prepectoral position
- Ventricular lead positioned in right ventricular apex position (arrow 1)
- Atrial lead positioned in right atrial appendage position (arrow 2)

Fig. 4.29

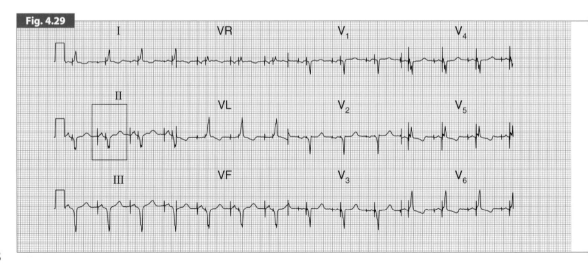

DUAL-CHAMBER PACEMAKERS (DDD)

DDD pacemakers are frequently used devices with two leads, one implanted in the right atrium and one in the right ventricle (Fig. 4.28).

The right atrial and ventricular chambers are both sensed. The atrial pacing lead will pace if no atrial activity is sensed within a predetermined interval. A maximum PR interval is also predetermined. If this is exceeded (following either a spontaneous P wave or a paced P wave) and no ventricular beat is sensed, then the ventricular paced beat is triggered.

Dual-chamber pacing is appropriate with the conditions listed in Box 4.7.

ECG APPEARANCE

When both the atrium and the ventricle are being paced, an atrial pacing spike is followed by a paced P wave, then a ventricular pacing spike is followed by a paced ventricular beat (Fig. 4.29).

When the intrinsic atrial rate exceeds the threshold for atrial pacing, 'atrial tracking' occurs. Atrial sensing takes place, but the intrinsic PR interval is longer than the programmed AV delay – leading to ventricular pacing. The ECG shows no atrial pacing spikes, but shows spontaneous P waves followed by ventricular pacing spikes and paced ventricular beats (Fig. 4.30).

Box 4.7 **Indications for dual-chamber pacing**

- Mobitz type II second degree heart block
- Third degree heart block
- Bradycardia–tachycardia syndrome

DDD pacing: atrial and ventricular pacing
Note
- Continuous atrial and ventricular pacing throughout
- Pacing spikes precede both P waves and QRS complexes

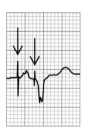

Atrial pacing followed by ventricular pacing in lead II

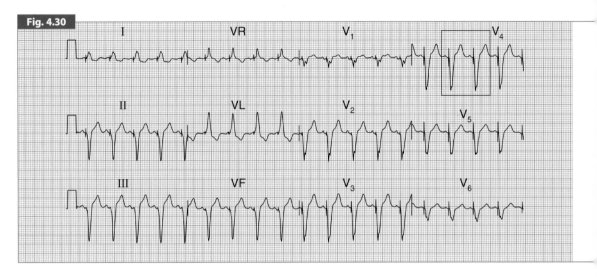

Fig. 4.30

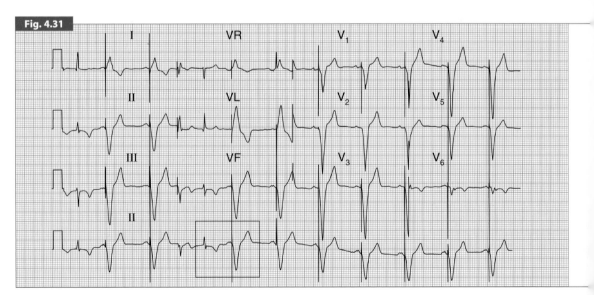

Fig. 4.31

DDD pacing: atrial tracking

Note
- Atrial sensing and ventricular pacing
- Non-paced P waves are followed by ventricular pacing spikes and paced ventricular complexes

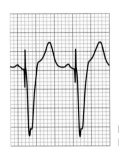

Pacing spike following
P wave in lead V$_4$

DDD pacing: intermittent

Note
- Atrial tracking, with atrial sensing and ventricular pacing
- The first, fourth and fifth QRS complexes show the intrinsic underlying rhythm, with appropriate ventricular sensing
- Large pacing spikes are consistent with a unipolar ventricular lead

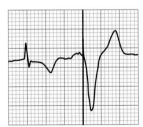

Intrinsic beat followed by a
beat showing atrial sensing
and ventricular pacing

Atrial pacing with ventricular tracking would be an unusual but theoretically possible situation. It would occur if the intrinsic atrial rate was slower than the threshold for atrial pacing, but the PR interval was shorter than the programmed AV delay. Hence there would be atrial pacing and intrinsic QRS complexes. The ECG would show atrial pacing spikes, paced P waves and spontaneous conducted ventricular beats.

In intermittent pacing, spontaneous atrial or ventricular activity will be sensed – leading to the inhibition of pacing in that chamber. If the programmed maximum PR interval is not exceeded, sensed atrial contraction may be followed by an AV conducted beat and a sensed QRS complex. The ECG will then show some intrinsic rhythm and some intermittent pacing (Fig. 4.31).

SPECIALIST FUNCTIONS

Rate response (DDDR) pacing allows an increase in pacing rate to a preset higher level in the presence of increased activity, allowing some increase in the heart rate with exercise.

Anti-AF algorithms trigger atrial pacing if atrial activity is sensed at a high rate, suggesting the onset of atrial arrhythmia. The aim is to control the atria at a lower rate.

ABNORMAL PACEMAKER FUNCTION

Pacemaker failure is rare. Most failures are due to problems with the pacing and/or sensing functions of the device. Complete diagnosis will usually require remote interrogation of the pacemaker, by placing over the implanted device a wand or header connected to a specialist programmer. This reveals information about how the device has been performing, as well as assessment of the leads and pacemaker function. There are various potential causes of device failure. Early after implantation, lead displacement may occur (Fig. 4.32). Rarer causes include lead insulation failure or lead fracture (Fig. 4.33). Unexpected battery depletion is rare, because devices are usually monitored regularly.

The investigation of pacemaker malfunction requires specialist techniques and expertise, and the 12-lead ECG can be extremely helpful in showing what has gone wrong.

FAILED PACING CAPTURE

This occurs when the voltage delivered to the pacemaker lead fails to trigger myocardial depolarization. It is characterized by the presence of pacing spikes but no subsequent atrial or ventricular depolarization (Figs 4.34 and 4.35).

Fig. 4.32

Chest X-ray showing right atrial and ventricular lead displacement

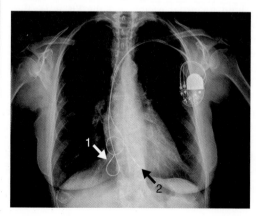

Note
- Compare with Figure 4.28
- The right atrial lead has been displaced from the atrial appendage, to a position much lower in the right atrium (arrow 1)
- The right ventricular lead is looped in the right atrium, with the tip displaced from the apex of the right ventricle (arrow 2)
- Atrial and ventricular pacing and sensing were lost in this patient

Fig. 4.33

Chest X-ray showing fractured pacing lead

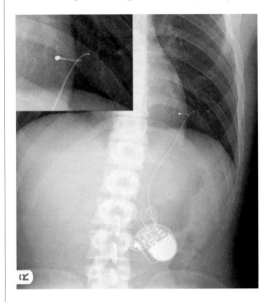

Note
- Abdominally placed pacemaker unit (in a child)
- Epicardial lead placed on the epicardial surface of the heart rather than within the right ventricle (endocardial)
- Fracture of the lead just proximal to the lead tip (enlarged inset)

UNDER-SENSING

'Under-sensing' occurs when the device develops an inability to detect intrinsic cardiac activity, and thus fails to suppress pacing in response to an intrinsic beat. The ECG is characterized by the presence of paced and normal beats closer together than would be expected from the programmed interval (Figs 4.36 and 4.37).

OVER-SENSING OR FAR-FIELD SENSING

This arises when sensing occurs in the absence of real intrinsic cardiac activity, triggering the inappropriate suppression of pacing. The ECG is characterized by inappropriately long intervals between beats, when pacing would be expected (Fig. 4.38).

PACEMAKER-MEDIATED TACHYCARDIA

A rare problem occurs when ventricular pacing triggers retrogradely conducted atrial depolarization, which is then sensed and triggers further ventricular pacing at an inappropriately short interval (Fig. 4.39). Pacemakers have a function for preventing this, called PVARP (post-ventricular atrial refractory period). This is a refractory period after ventricular pacing, in which atrial activity cannot be sensed. Inappropriately rapid pacing will require specialist assessment.

203

Fig. 4.34

Failed pacemaker capture

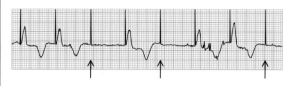

Note
- Intermittent failed right ventricular capture – pacing spikes (arrowed) not followed by a QRS complex (VVI pacemaker; no underlying cardiac rhythm)

Fig. 4.35

Failed pacemaker capture
Redrawn by permission of Medtronic

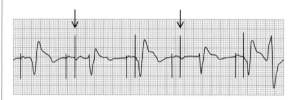

Note
- Intermittent failed right ventricular capture (arrowed)
- Ventricular sensing and atrial function appear normal (DDD pacemaker)

Fig. 4.36

Pacemaker under-sensing

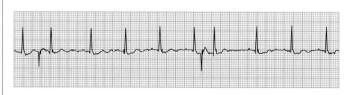

Note
- Atrial under-sensing (AAI pacemaker)
- Inappropriate atrial pacing spikes, which capture and conduct from atria to ventricles despite an adequate rate of intrinsic atrial activity – indicating failed atrial sensing

Fig. 4.37

Pacemaker under-sensing
Redrawn by permission of Medtronic

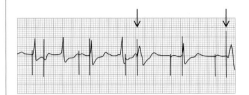

Note
- Ventricular under-sensing (DDD pacemaker)
- Atrial and ventricular pacing spikes occur despite an underlying rhythm, indicating failed sensing
- The third and fifth ventricular pacing spikes are normally conducted (arrowed). The remainder form fusion complexes, between the paced and intrinsic QRS complexes

Fig. 4.38

Pacemaker over-sensing
Redrawn by permission of Medtronic

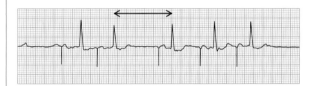

Note
- There is an inappropriate gap between the paced atrial and tracked ventricular complexes (arrowed). This could be due to atrial or ventricular over-sensing. In this case the ventricular lead was at fault.

Fig. 4.39

Pacemaker-mediated tachycardia
Redrawn by permission of Medtronic

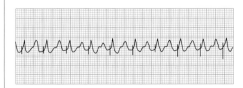

Note
- Tachyarrhythmia with pacing spike preceding each QRS complex

MAGNET RATE

A simple check of pacemaker function can be made by applying a magnet to the skin over the device. This will trigger obligate pacing at the 'magnet rate' (Fig. 4.40). Pacing spikes will be delivered at this fixed preset rate regardless of the intrinsic rhythm, and should cause depolarization unless delivered at the time of an intrinsic beat, when fusion may occur. The pacemaker will return to normal programmed function when the magnet is removed.

INDICATIONS FOR PACEMAKER INSERTION

Table 4.2 summarizes the situations in which permanent pacing is indicated.

Fig. 4.40

Magnet pacing – DDD pacemaker

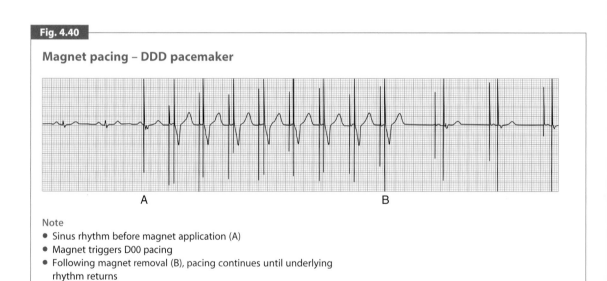

A   B

Note
- Sinus rhythm before magnet application (A)
- Magnet triggers D00 pacing
- Following magnet removal (B), pacing continues until underlying rhythm returns

---

Table 4.2 **Types of device and clinical indications**

Device function	Chamber(s) with implanted electrode	Clinical indications
Single chamber		
VVI	Right ventricle	Slow atrial fibrillation, or atrial fibrillation with pauses 'Backup' with sinus node disease or atrioventricular block Bradycardia–tachycardia syndrome Very elderly patients
AAI	Right atrium	Sinus node disease without atrioventricular block Carotid sinus syncope
VVI/ICD	Right ventricle	Survived cardiac arrest due to ventricular fibrillation or ventricular tachycardia (VT) Spontaneous sustained VT causing syncope or haemodynamic compromise Sustained VT or cardiac arrest and ejection fraction < 35% with symptoms no worse than NYHA Class III* Familial risk of sudden cardiac death (HCM (hypertrophic cardiomyopathy), long QT syndrome, Brugada syndrome, ARVD (arrhythmogenic right ventricular dysplasia)) Surgical repair of congenital heart disease Non-sustained VT and ejection fraction < 35% with symptoms no worse than NYHA Class III*, plus a history of myocardial infarction (> 4 weeks old) and VT inducible by electrophysiology Ejection fraction < 30% and QRS complex >120 ms, and no myocardial infarction in the previous 4 weeks
Dual chamber		
DDD	Right ventricle Right atrium	Atrioventricular block, usually third degree block or Mobitz type II second degree block Bradycardia–tachycardia syndrome
DDD/ICD	Right ventricle – shocking lead Right atrium – pacing lead	Indications as for VVI/ICD but in patient requiring DDD pacemaker function
Biventricular		
CRT	Right ventricle Left ventricle via coronary sinus ± Right atrium	NYHA Class III* or IV* heart failure and ejection fraction < 35%, plus either left bundle branch block with QRS complexes > 150 ms, or QRS complexes 120–150 ms with echocardiographic dyssynchrony
CRTD	Right ventricle – shocking lead Coronary sinus – left ventricular pacing lead ± Right atrial pacing lead	Indications as for CRT and ICD Patient groups benefiting from combined device not yet clearly defined

* New York Heart Association Functional Classification; Class III/IV indicates moderate/severe heart failure.

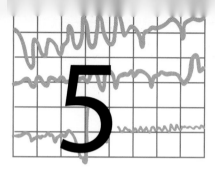

5 The ECG in patients with chest pain

History and examination	**209**
Acute chest pain	209
Chronic chest pain	211
The ECG in the presence of chest pain	212
The ECG in patients with myocardial ischaemia	**212**
ECG changes in ST segment elevation myocardial infarction (STEMI)	214
ECG changes in non-ST segment elevation myocardial infarction (NSTEMI)	241
Ischaemia without myocardial infarction	241
The ECG in pulmonary embolism	**247**
The ECG in other causes of chest pain	**251**
Pericarditis	251
Aortic stenosis and aortic dissection	251
ECG pitfalls in the diagnosis of chest pain	**252**
R wave changes	255
ST segment and T wave changes	256
What to do	**264**
Acute chest pain suggesting myocardial infarction	264
Other investigations for patients with acute chest pain	264
The investigation of chronic chest pain	265
Exercise testing	270
Management of chest pain	285

HISTORY AND EXAMINATION

There are many causes of chest pain. All the non-cardiac conditions can mimic a myocardial infarction, and so the ECG can be extremely useful when making a diagnosis. However, the ECG is less important than the history and (to a lesser extent) the physical examination, because the ECG can be normal in the first few hours of a myocardial infarction.

Some causes of chest pain are listed in Box 5.1.

The ECG in Figure 5.1 was recorded in an A & E department from a 44-year-old man with rather vague chest pain. He was thought to have a viral illness and his ECG was considered to be within normal limits. He was allowed home, and died later that day. The post-mortem examination showed a myocardial infarction which was probably a few hours old, and corresponded with his A & E attendance.

ACUTE CHEST PAIN

The features of acute chest pain associated with different causes are summarized in Box 5.2.

The physical examination of a patient with chest pain may reveal nothing other than the signs associated with the pain itself (anxiety, sinus tachycardia, restlessness or a cold and sweaty skin), but some specific signs are worth looking for:

- Left ventricular failure suggests myocardial infarction.
- A raised jugular venous pressure suggests myocardial infarction or pulmonary embolus.
- A pleural friction rub suggests pulmonary embolism or infection.
- A pericardial friction rub suggests pericarditis (?viral, ?secondary to myocardial infarction) or aortic dissection.
- Aortic regurgitation suggests aortic dissection.
- Unequal pulses or blood pressure in the arms suggests aortic dissection.
- Bony tenderness suggests musculoskeletal pain.

Box 5.1 **Causes of chest pain**

Acute chest pain	Chronic or recurrent chest pain
• Myocardial infarction • Pulmonary embolism • Pneumothorax • Other causes of pleuritic pain • Pericarditis • Aortic dissection • Ruptured oesophagus • Oesophagitis • Collapsed vertebra • Herpes zoster	• Angina • Nerve root pain • Muscular pain • Oesophageal reflux • Nonspecific pain

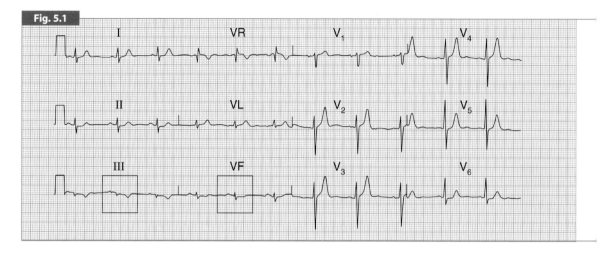

Fig. 5.1

Box 5.2 Features of acute chest pain

Myocardial infarction
- Central
- Radiates to neck, jaw, teeth, arm(s) or back
- Severe
- Associated with nausea, vomiting and sweating
- Not all patients have typical pain, and pain can even be absent

Pulmonary embolism
- Pain similar to myocardial infarction if the embolus is central
- Pleuritic pain if the embolus is peripheral
- Associated with breathlessness or haemoptysis
- Can cause haemodynamic collapse

Other lung disease, e.g. infection or pneumothorax
- Pleuritic
  — worse on breathing
  — often associated with a cough

Pericardial pain
- Can mimic both cardiac ischaemia and pleuritic pain
- Can be recognized because it is relieved by sitting up and leaning forward

Aortic dissection
- Typically causes a 'tearing' pain (as opposed to the 'crushing' sensation of a myocardial infarction)
- Usually radiates to the back

Oesophageal rupture
- Follows vomiting

Spinal pain
- Affected by posture
- Associated root pain follows the nerve root distribution

Shingles (herpes zoster)
- Catches everyone out until the rash appears
- Tenderness of the skin may provide a clue

Nonspecific ST segment/T wave changes

Note

- Sinus rhythm
- Normal axis
- Normal QRS complexes
- ST segments probably normal, though possibly depressed in leads III and VF
- T wave inverted in lead III (possibly a normal variant) and flattened in VF

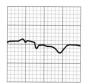

Inverted T wave
in lead III

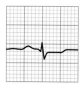

Flattened T wave
in lead VF

CHRONIC CHEST PAIN

The main differential diagnosis of chronic chest pain is between angina and the chest pain that is common in middle-aged men, but for which no clear diagnosis is usually made. This pain is sometimes called 'atypical chest pain', but this is a dangerous diagnostic label because it implies that there is a diagnosis (by implication, cardiac ischaemia) but that the symptoms are 'atypical'. Some of these pains are musculoskeletal, Tietze's syndrome of pain from the costochondral junctions being the most obvious, but in most cases the best diagnostic label is 'chest pain of unknown cause'. This indicates a possible need for later re-evaluation.

The important features in the history that point to a diagnosis of angina are that the pain:

- is predictable
- usually occurs after a constant amount of exercise
- is worse in cold or windy weather
- is induced by emotional stress
- is induced by sexual intercourse
- is relieved by rest, and rapidly relieved by a short-acting nitrate.

The physical signs to look for are:

- evidence of risk factors (high blood pressure, cholesterol deposits, signs of smoking)
- any signs of cardiac disease (aortic stenosis, an enlarged heart, signs of heart failure)
- anaemia (which will exacerbate myocardial ischaemia)
- signs of peripheral vascular disease (which would suggest that coronary disease is also present).

THE ECG IN THE PRESENCE OF CHEST PAIN

Remember that the ECG can be normal in the early stages of a myocardial infarction. Having said that:

- An abnormal ECG is usually necessary to make a diagnosis of myocardial infarction before treatment is started.
- An ECG will demonstrate ischaemia in patients with angina *provided that* the patient has pain at the time the ECG is recorded.
- With pulmonary embolism there may be classical ECG changes, but these are often not present.
- With pericarditis, ECG changes, if present at all, are very nonspecific.

THE ECG IN PATIENTS WITH MYOCARDIAL ISCHAEMIA

Myocardial infarction is, properly, a term describing myocardial cell death due to ischaemia. The histological changes – and ECG changes – can take several hours to appear, and the entire process leading to a healed infarction can take 5 or 6 weeks. Myocardial injury causes release into the blood of biomarkers such as troponin T or I and the MB fraction of creatine kinase, CK-MB. Therefore the release of these biomarkers can reflect the necrosis of myocardial cells, but it also occurs in situations other than coronary artery occlusion (Box 5.3). Thus, although a rise in the blood levels of biomarkers supports the diagnosis of myocardial infarction it is not sufficient, and the most commonly used parts of the 'universal definition' of myocardial infarction, require both clinical evidence of myocardial ischaemia and a rise and/or fall of blood troponin levels. Box 5.4 shows the types of infarction listed in the universal definition, drawn up by the ESC/ACCF/AHA/WHF Task Force (Jaffe, A.S., Simoons, M.L., Chaitman, B.R. and White, H.D., on behalf of the Joint ESC/ACCF/AHA/WHF Task Force for the Universal Definition of Myocardial Infarction. *European Heart Journal* (2012) 33, 2551–2567). Box 5.5 lists the diagnostic criteria for each type of infarction.

The universal definition does not use the term 'acute coronary syndrome' at all, although this is a term in widespread clinical use, albeit with variations in what should be included. The term is most commonly used to describe patients with a clinical 'coronary event' of various types, including:

Box 5.3 Causes of plasma troponin elevation other than myocardial infarction

- Extreme exertion
- Trauma
- Congestive heart failure (acute or chronic)
- Aortic dissection
- Aortic valve disease
- Hypertrophic cardiomyopathy
- Arrhythmias, including heart block
- Apical ballooning syndrome
- Rhabdomyolysis following cardiac injury
- Pulmonary embolism
- Renal failure
- Stroke; subarachnoid haemorrhage
- Infiltrative diseases (e.g. amyloid, sarcoid)
- Inflammatory diseases – myocarditis and pericarditis
- Drug toxicity
- Critically ill patients with respiratory failure or sepsis
- Burns

Box 5.4 Types of myocardial infarction

1. Spontaneous myocardial infarction, due to plaque rupture and coronary artery occlusion due to thrombosis
2. Myocardial infarction secondary to ischaemia imbalance (e.g. coronary spasm, embolism, arrhythmias, hypotension)
3. Myocardial infarction resulting in death when biomarker values are not available (suggestive symptoms with ECG changes)
4. Myocardial infarction related to percutaneous coronary intervention (PCI). Type 4b is infarction related to stent thrombosis
5. Myocardial infarction related to coronary artery bypass grafting (CABG)

Box 5.5 Criteria for myocardial infarction

Acute myocardial infarction
- Detection of rise and/or fall of cardiac biomarkers (preferably troponin) together with evidence of myocardial ischaemia and at least one of the following:
  — symptoms of ischaemia
  — ECG – new changes in ST segments or T waves, or new left bundle branch block
  — development of pathological Q waves
  — imaging evidence of new loss of viable myocardium or new regional wall motion abnormality
- Sudden unexpected cardiac death, often with symptoms and ECG changes of ischaemia; or evidence of fresh coronary thrombus at post mortem, before blood samples are taken or before a rise in cardiac biomarkers could be expected
- Myocardial infarction related to PCI (percutaneous coronary intervention) – a rise of troponin to five times the upper limit of normal, plus new ischaemic symptoms or new ECG changes or imaging evidence of loss of viable myocardium
- Myocardial infarction related to CABG (coronary artery bypass grafting) – elevation of troponin level to ten times the upper limit of normal, plus either new ECG changes, evidence of loss of viable myocardium, or angiographically demonstrated graft occlusion
- Pathological findings of an acute infarction

Prior myocardial infarction
Any one of:
- Pathological Q waves, with or without symptoms
- Imaging evidence of loss of viable myocardium
- Pathological findings of healed or healing infarction

- chest pain with ischaemic ST segment depression but no troponin rise (what used to be called 'unstable angina')
- chest pain with a troponin rise and T wave inversion or ST segment depression (non-ST segment elevation myocardial infarction, NSTEMI)
- chest pain with a troponin rise and ST segment elevation (ST segment elevation myocardial infarction, STEMI)

and sometimes

- sudden death due to coronary disease, without a troponin rise or ECG evidence.

'Stable angina' is an entirely proper diagnostic label for a patient with intermittent chest pain associated with transient ECG changes, and 'chest pain of unknown cause' is the best label if no diagnosis has been made.

ECG CHANGES IN ST SEGMENT ELEVATION MYOCARDIAL INFARCTION (STEMI)

The sequence of features characteristic of STEMI is:

- normal ECG
- ST segment elevation
- development of Q waves
- ST segment returns to the baseline
- T waves become inverted.

The universal definition of STEMI requires new ST segment elevation at the J point (the junction of the S wave and the ST segment) in two contiguous leads, with the cut-off points in leads V_2–V_3 at > 0.3 mV in men or > 0.15 mV in women, and in other leads at > 0.1 mV. The ECG leads that show the changes typical of a myocardial infarction depend on the part of the heart affected.

Fig. 5.2

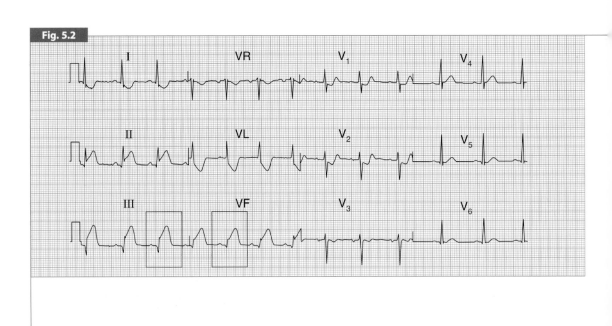

INFERIOR INFARCTION

Figures 5.2, 5.3 and 5.4 show traces taken from a patient with a typical history of myocardial infarction: on admission to hospital, 3 h later, and 2 days later. The main changes are in the inferior leads: II, III and VF. Here the ST segments are initially raised, but then Q waves appear and the T waves become inverted. Figure 5.2 includes coronary angiograms showing the effects of an occluded right coronary artery in an inferior STEMI.

Acute inferior infarction

Note

- Sinus rhythm
- Normal axis
- Small Q waves in leads II–III, VF
- Raised ST segments in leads II–III, VF
- Depressed ST segments in leads I, VL, V_2–V_3
- Inverted T waves in leads I, VL, V_3

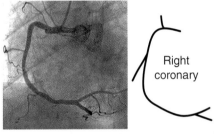

Right coronary

Angiogram showing normal right coronary artery

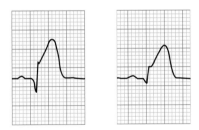

Raised ST segments in leads III and VF

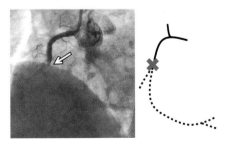

Angiogram showing occluded right coronary artery in inferior STEMI

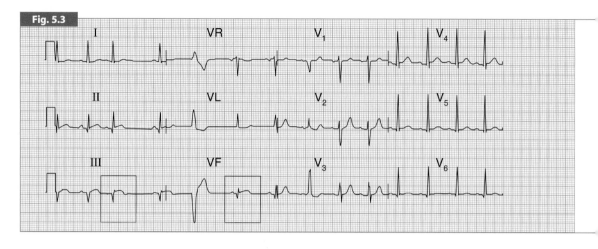

Fig. 5.3

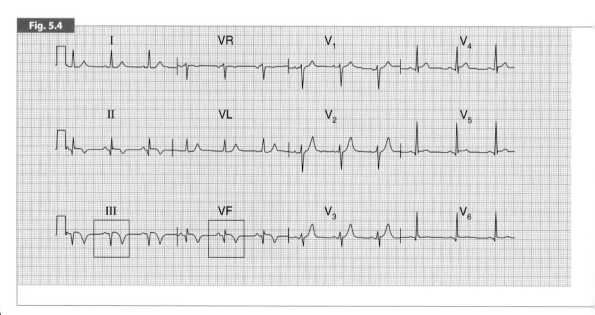

Fig. 5.4

Evolving inferior infarction

Note
- Same patient as in Figures 5.2 and 5.4
- Sinus rhythm with ventricular extrasystoles
- Normal axis
- Deeper Q waves in leads II–III, VF
- ST segments returning to normal, but still elevated in inferior leads
- Less ST segment depression in leads I, VL, V₃

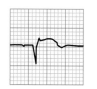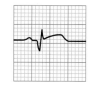

Deeper Q waves in leads III and VF

Evolving inferior infarction

Note
- Same patient as in Figures 5.2 and 5.3
- Sinus rhythm
- Normal axis
- Q waves in leads II–III, VF
- ST segments nearly back to normal
- T wave inversion in leads II–III, VF
- Lateral ischaemia has cleared (as shown by ST segments in lateral leads)

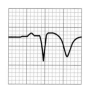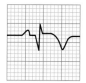

Q waves, normal ST segments, and inverted T waves in leads III and VF

ANTERIOR AND LATERAL INFARCTION

The changes of anterior infarction are seen in leads V₂–V₅. Lead V₁, which lies over the right ventricle, is seldom affected (see Fig. 5.5, which includes corresponding coronary angiograms).

When the lateral wall of the left ventricle is damaged by occlusion of the left circumflex coronary artery, leads I, VL and V₆ will show infarction changes. Figure 5.6 shows the record of a patient with an acute lateral STEMI, with the corresponding coronary angiograms. Figure 5.7 shows a record taken 3 days after a lateral infarction, with Q waves and inverted T waves in leads I, VL and V₆.

The ECG in Figure 5.8 shows an acute STEMI affecting both the anerior and lateral parts of the left ventricle.

Fig. 5.5

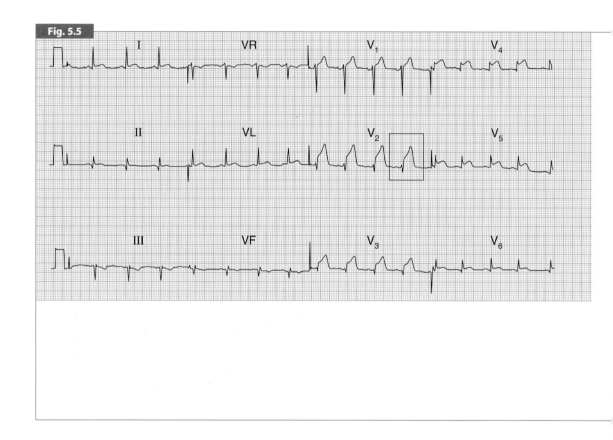

Anterior infarction

Note
- Sinus rhythm
- Normal axis
- Raised ST segments in leads V_2–V_5

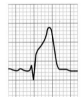

Raised ST segment in lead V_2

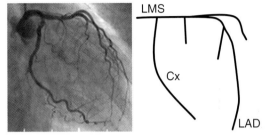

Angiogram showing normal left coronary artery:
  LMS – left main stem coronary artery
  Cx – circumflex branch
  LAD – left anterior descending branch

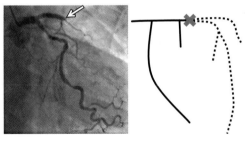

Angiogram showing occluded left anterior descending branch in anterior STEMI

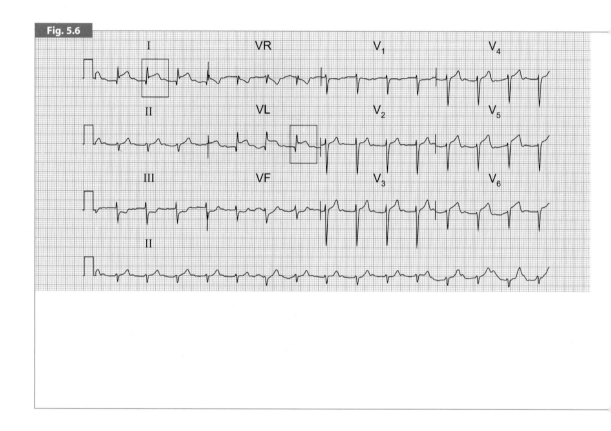

Fig. 5.6

Acute lateral infarction

Note

- Sinus rhythm
- First degree block
- Left axis deviation
- Normal axis
- Q waves in leads I, VL
- Raised ST segments in leads I, VL, V_5–V_6

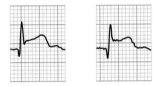

Raised ST segments in leads I and VL

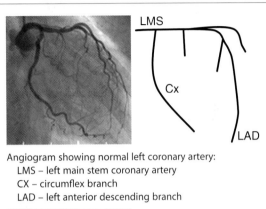

Angiogram showing normal left coronary artery:
   LMS – left main stem coronary artery
   CX – circumflex branch
   LAD – left anterior descending branch

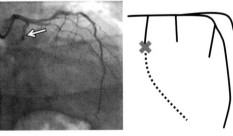

Angiogram showing occluded left circumflex branch in lateral STEMI

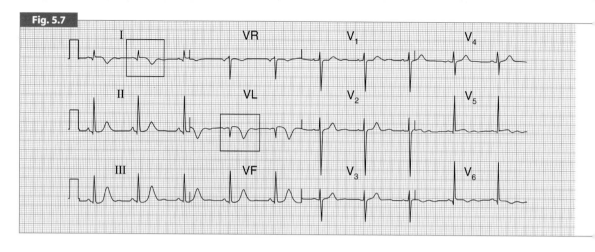

Fig. 5.7

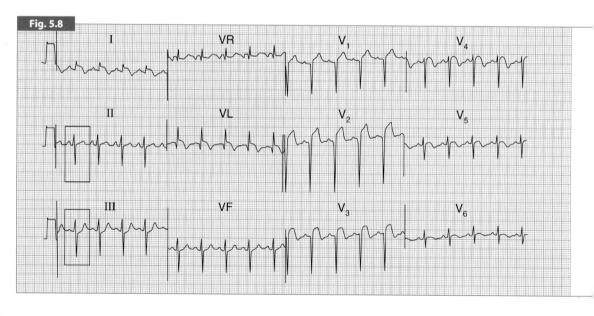

Fig. 5.8

Lateral infarction (after 3 days)

Note

- Sinus rhythm
- Normal axis
- Q waves in leads I, VL, ?V_6 (could be septal)
- ST segments isoelectric
- Inverted T waves in leads I, VL, V_6

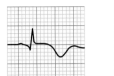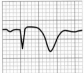

Inverted T waves in leads I and VL

Acute anterolateral infarction with left axis deviation

Note

- Sinus rhythm
- Left axis deviation
- ST segments now returning to normal
- T wave inversion in leads I, VL, V_4–V_5

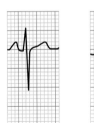

S waves in leads II and III: left axis deviation

223

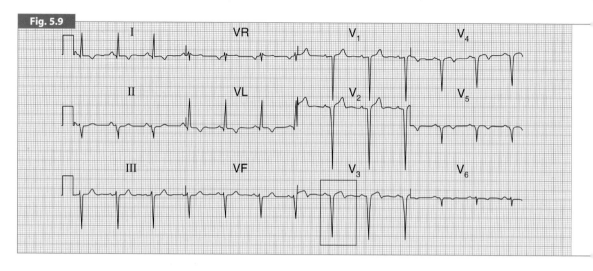

Fig. 5.9

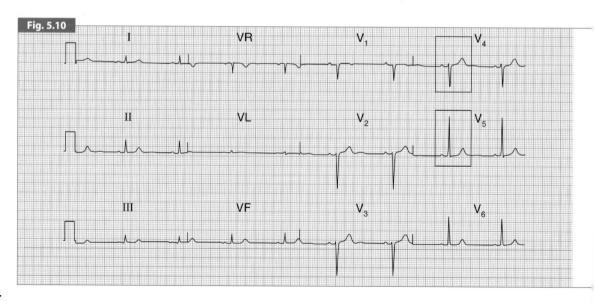

Fig. 5.10

Anterolateral infarction, ?age

Note

- Sinus rhythm
- Left axis deviation
- Q waves in leads I–II, V_2–V_5
- Raised ST segments in leads V_3–V_5
- Inverted T waves in leads I, VL, V_4–V_6

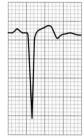

Raised ST segment in lead V_3

Old anterior infarction

Note

- Sinus rhythm
- Normal axis
- Small R waves in leads V_3–V_4, large R waves in V_5: this is 'poor R wave progression'

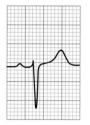 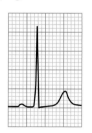

Small R wave in lead V_4 Tall R wave in lead V_5

The ECG in Figure 5.9 was recorded several weeks after an anterolateral myocardial infarction. Although the changes in leads I and VL appear 'old', having an isoelectric ST segment, there is still ST segment elevation in leads V_3–V_5. If the patient had just been admitted to hospital with chest pain these changes would be taken to indicate an acute infarction, but this patient had had pain more than a month previously. Persistent ST segment elevation is quite common after an anterior infarction: it sometimes indicates the development of a left ventricular aneurysm, but it is not reliable evidence of this.

An old anterior infarction often causes only what is called 'poor R wave progression'. Figure 5.10 shows the record from a patient who had had an anterior infarction some years previously. A normal ECG would show a progressive increase in the size of the R wave from lead V_1 to V_5 or V_6. In this case the R wave remains very small in leads V_3 and V_4, but becomes normal-sized in V_5. This loss of 'progression' indicates the old infarction.

The time taken for the various ECG changes of infarction to occur is extremely variable, and the ECG is an unreliable way of deciding when an infarction occurred. Serial records showing progressive changes are the only way of timing the infarction from the ECG.

POSTERIOR INFARCTION

It is possible to 'look at' the back of the heart by placing the V lead on the back of the left side of the chest, but this is not done routinely because it is inconvenient and the complexes recorded are often small.

An infarction of the posterior wall of the left ventricle can, however, be detected from the ordinary 12-lead ECG because it causes a dominant R wave in lead V_1. Normally the left ventricle, being more muscular than the right, exerts a greater influence on the ECG, so in lead V_1 the QRS complex is predominantly downward. With a posterior infarction, the rearward-moving electrical forces are lost, so lead V_1 'sees' the unopposed forward-moving depolarization of the right ventricle, and records a predominantly upright QRS complex.

Fig. 5.11

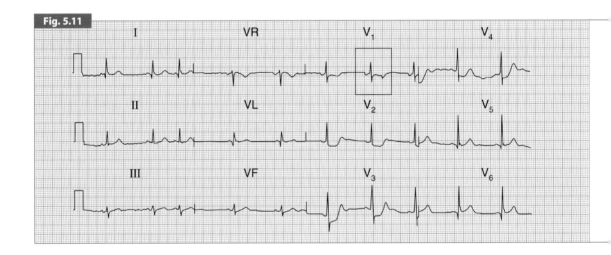

Figure 5.11 shows the first record from a patient with acute chest pain. There is a dominant R wave in lead V_1 and ischaemic ST segment depression (see p. 231) in leads V_2–V_4. The chest electrodes were then moved to the V_7–V_9 positions: all in the same horizontal plane as V_5, with V_7 on the posterior axillary line, V_9 at the edge of the spine, and V_8 halfway between, on the midscapular line. The ECG record then showed raised ST segments, with Q waves typical of an acute infarction.

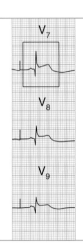

Posterior infarction

Note

- Sinus rhythm with atrial extrasystoles
- Normal axis
- Dominant R waves in lead V_1 suggest posterior infarction
- ST segment depression in leads V_2–V_4
- Q waves and ST segment elevation in leads V_7–V_9 (posterior leads)

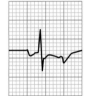

Dominant R wave in lead V_1

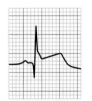

Q wave and raised ST segment in lead V_7

RIGHT VENTRICULAR INFARCTION

Inferior infarction is sometimes associated with infarction of the right ventricle. Clinically, this is suspected in a patient with an inferior infarction when the lungs are clear but the jugular venous pressure is elevated. The ECG will show raised ST segments in leads recorded from the right side of the heart. The positions of the leads correspond to those on the left side as follows: V_1R is in the normal V_2 position; V_2R is in the normal V_1 position; V_3R etc. are on the right side, in positions corresponding to V_3 etc. on the left side. Figure 5.12 is from a patient with an acute right ventricular infarct.

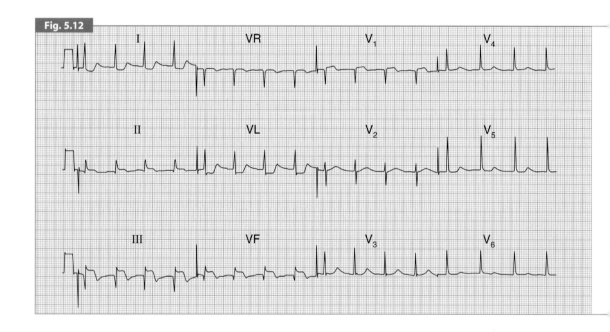

Fig. 5.12

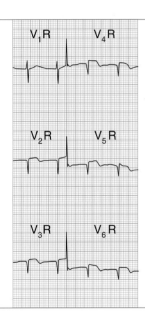

Inferior and right ventricular infarction
Note
- Sinus rhythm
- Normal axis
- Raised ST segments in leads II–III, VF
- Raised ST segments in leads V_2R–V_5R
- Q waves in leads III, VF, V_2R–V_6R

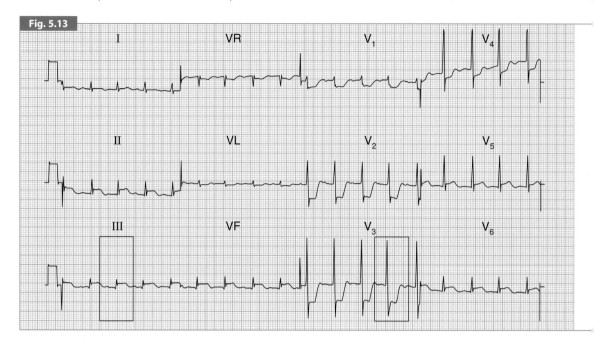

Fig. 5.13

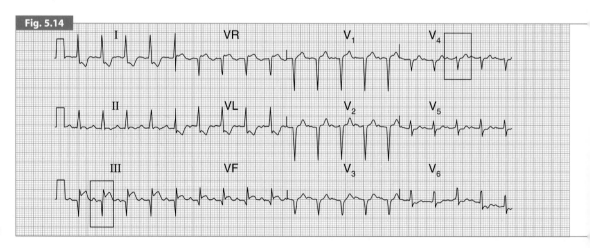

Fig. 5.14

Acute inferior infarction and anterior ischaemia

Note

- Sinus rhythm
- Normal axis
- Raised ST segments in leads II–III, VF
- ST segment depression in leads V_1–V_4

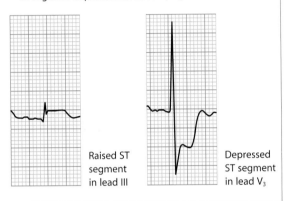

Raised ST segment in lead III

Depressed ST segment in lead V_3

MULTIPLE INFARCTIONS

Infarction of more than one part of the left ventricle causes changes in several different ECG territories. This usually implies disease in more than one of the main coronary arteries. The ECG in Figure 5.13 shows an acute inferior myocardial infarction and marked anterior ST segment depression. Later, coronary angiography showed that this patient had a significant stenosis of the left main coronary artery.

Figure 5.14 is the record from a patient with an acute inferior myocardial infarction. Poor R wave progression in leads V_2–V_4 indicates an old anterior infarction as well.

Figure 5.15 is an ECG showing an acute inferior STEMI and anterior T wave inversion due to an NSTEMI of uncertain age.

Figure 5.16 is an ECG showing an acute anterior myocardial infarction. Deep Q waves in leads III and VF indicate an old inferior infarction.

Acute inferior and old anterior infarctions

Note

- Sinus rhythm
- Normal axis
- Q waves in leads III, VF
- Raised ST segments in leads III, VF
- Poor R wave progression in anterior leads

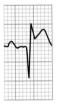
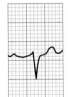

Q wave and raised ST segment in lead III

Loss of R wave in lead V_4

231

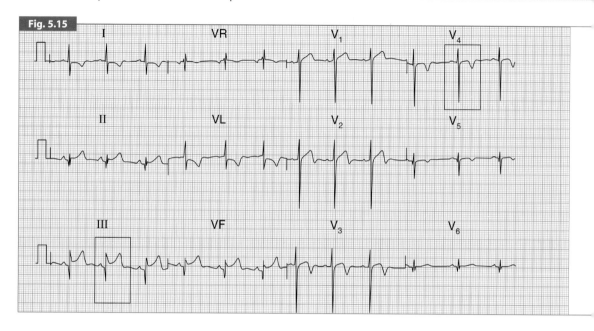

Fig. 5.15

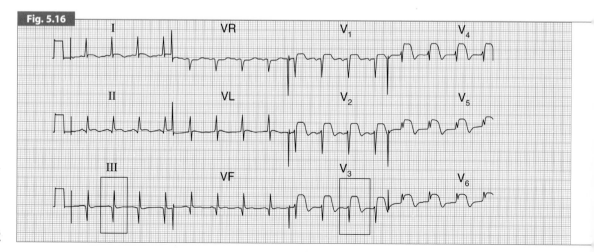

Fig. 5.16

Acute inferior infarction (STEMI) and anterior NSTEMI

Note
- Sinus rhythm
- Normal axis
- Q waves in leads II–III, VF
- ST segment elevation in leads II–III, VF
- T wave inversion in leads V_3–V_5

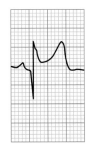

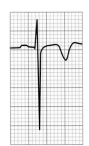

Q wave and ST segment elevation in lead III

Inverted T wave in lead V_4

Acute anterior and old inferior infarctions

Note
- Sinus rhythm
- Normal axis
- Q waves in leads II–III, VF
- ST segment elevation in leads V_2–V_6

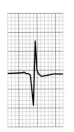

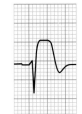

Q wave in lead III

Raised ST segment in lead V_3

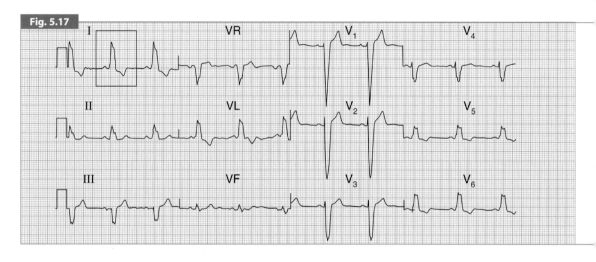

Fig. 5.17

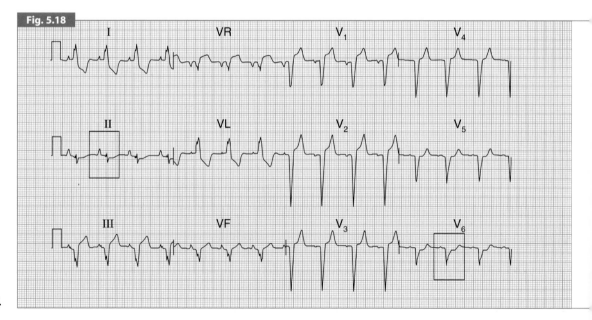

Fig. 5.18

Left bundle branch block

Note
- Sinus rhythm
- Normal axis
- Wide QRS complexes with LBBB pattern
- Inverted T waves in leads I, VL, V$_5$–V$_6$

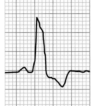

Broad QRS complex and inverted T wave in lead I

Left bundle branch block, ?right ventricular overload

Note
- Sinus rhythm
- Peaked P waves in leads I–II
- LBBB pattern, most obvious in leads I–II
- Persistent S wave in lead V$_6$

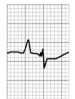
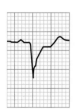

Peaked P wave in lead II

Persistent S wave in lead V$_6$

BUNDLE BRANCH BLOCK AND MYOCARDIAL INFARCTION

Left bundle branch block

Left bundle branch block (LBBB) is very rare in patients with totally normal hearts, but it may be associated with many different heart diseases (Box 5.6).

With LBBB, the abnormal and slow conduction in to the left ventricle, and the abnormal pattern of repolarization, mean that no changes due to myocardial infarction can be seen (Fig. 5.17). However, this does not mean that the ECG can be totally disregarded. If a patient has chest pain that could be ischaemic and the ECG shows LBBB that is known to be new, it can be assumed that an acute infarction has occurred and appropriate treatment should be given.

Figure 5.18 is the record from another patient presenting with chest pain who had LBBB, but there are important differences compared to Figure 5.17. Peaked P waves suggest right atrial hypertrophy. 'Clockwise rotation' with no left ventricular QRS complex pattern in lead V$_6$ raises the possibility of either a pulmonary embolus (see p. 247) or chronic lung disease.

Box 5.6 **Causes of left bundle branch block**

- Ischaemia
- Hypertension
- Cardiomyopathy
- Myocarditis
- Cardiac channelopathies
- Cardiac tumours
- Sarcoidosis
- Chagas disease
- Operated and unoperated congenital heart disease

Fig. 5.19

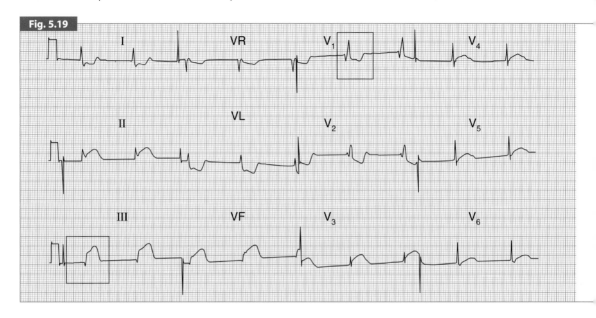

Fig. 5.20

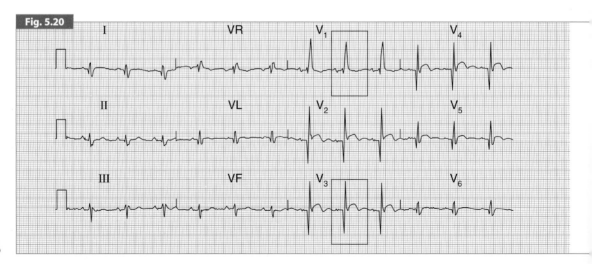

Right bundle branch block and acute inferior infarction

Note
- Sinus rhythm
- Normal axis
- Wide QRS complex with RSR^1 pattern in lead V$_1$
- Raised ST segments in leads II–III, VF

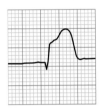 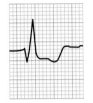

Raised ST segments in lead III

RSR^1 pattern in lead V$_1$

Right bundle branch block

Right bundle branch block (RBBB) will not necessarily obscure the pattern of inferior infarction (Fig. 5.19).

Anterior infarction is more difficult to detect, but RBBB does not affect the ST segment and when this is raised in a patient who clinically has had an infarction, the change is probably significant (Fig. 5.20).

ST segment depression associated with RBBB indicates ischaemia (Fig. 5.21). However, T wave inversion in the anterior leads (Fig. 5.22) is more difficult to interpret because it is a common feature of RBBB itself.

Right bundle branch block and anterior infarction

Note
- Sinus rhythm
- Normal axis
- RBBB pattern
- Raised ST segments in leads V$_2$–V$_5$

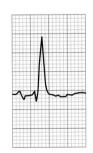 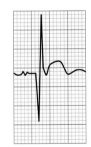

RSR^1 pattern in lead V$_1$

Raised ST segment in lead V$_3$

237

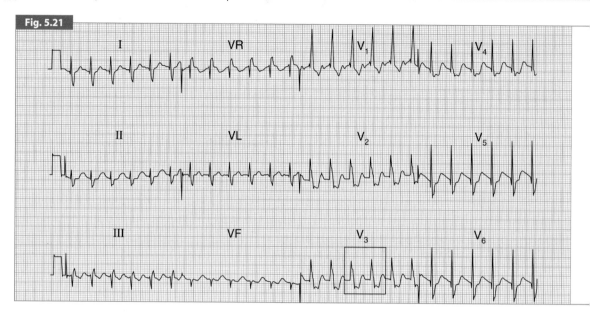

Fig. 5.21

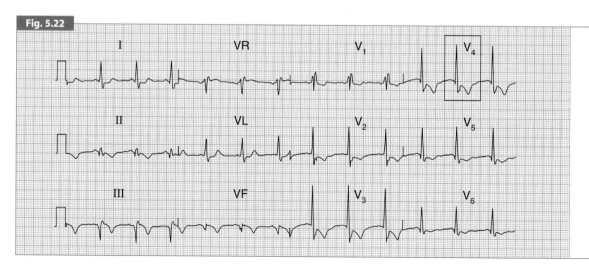

Fig. 5.22

Right bundle branch block and anterior ischaemia

Note
- Sinus rhythm
- RBBB pattern
- ST segment depression in leads V_2–V_4

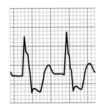

ST segment depression in lead V_3

Inferior infarction, right bundle branch block, ?anterior ischaemia

Note
- Sinus rhythm
- Q waves with inverted T waves in leads II–III, VF
- RBBB pattern
- Deep T wave inversion in leads V_3–V_4

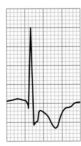

T wave inversion in lead V_4

239

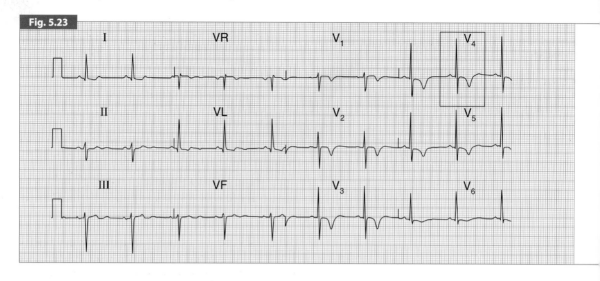

Fig. 5.23

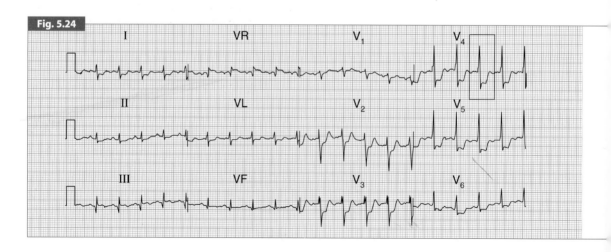

Fig. 5.24

Anterior non-ST segment elevation myocardial infarction (NSTEMI)

Note
- Sinus rhythm
- Left axis deviation
- Normal QRS complexes
- Inverted T waves in all chest leads

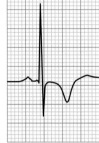

Inverted T wave in lead V$_4$

Anterior ischaemia, possible old inferior infarction

Note
- Sinus rhythm
- Normal axis
- Small Q waves in leads III, VF
- Inverted T waves in lead III
- Marked ST segment depression in leads V$_2$–V$_6$

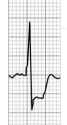

ST segment depression in lead V$_4$

ECG CHANGES IN NON-ST SEGMENT ELEVATION MYOCARDIAL INFARCTION (NSTEMI)

When the infarction does not involve the whole thickness of the ventricular wall, no electrical 'window' will be formed so there will be no Q waves: hence the term 'non-Q wave infarction', although this has now been superseded by the term 'NSTEMI'. The infarction causes an abnormality of repolarization that leads to T wave inversion. This pattern is most commonly seen in the anterior and lateral leads (Fig. 5.23).

This ECG pattern used to be called 'subendocardial infarction', but the pathological changes seen in heart muscle after myocardial infarction often do not fit neatly into 'subendocardial' or 'full thickness' patterns. Acute NSTEMI is usually associated with a rise in the blood troponin level. Compared with patients with STEMIs, those with NSTEMIs have a lower immediate fatality rate but a relatively high incidence of reinfarction during the following 3 months; thereafter their fatality rates are similar.

ISCHAEMIA WITHOUT MYOCARDIAL INFARCTION

Cardiac ischaemia causes horizontal ST segment depression; to be diagnostic of ischaemia, there must be horizontal or downward-sloping depression of > 0.05 mV in two contiguous leads, and/or T wave inversion of > 0.1 mV in two contiguous leads. Such changes appear and disappear with the pain of stable angina. Persistent pain and ST segment depression (Fig. 5.24) may not be associated with any rise in troponin level.

241

Fig. 5.25

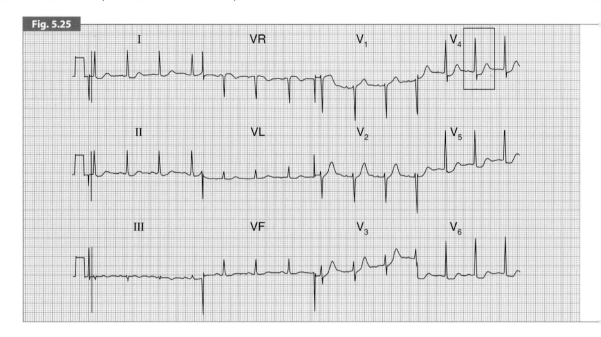

Fig. 5.26

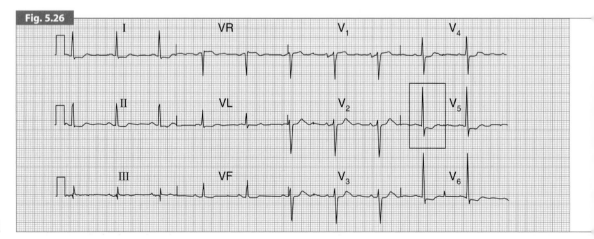

Anterior ischaemia

Note
- Sinus rhythm
- Normal axis
- Normal QRS complexes
- ST segment depression in leads V_4–V_6

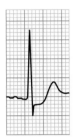

ST segment depression in lead V_4

If a patient has chest pain that persists long enough for him or her to seek hospital admission, and the ECG shows ST segment depression, the outlook is relatively poor – even when the depression is not marked (Figs 5.25 and 5.26) and there is no rise in troponin level. These patients usually need further investigation, though on the whole they can be managed as outpatients.

Ischaemia may be precipitated by an arrhythmia, and will be resolved when either the heart rate is controlled or the arrhythmia is corrected. The ECG in Figure 5.27 shows ischaemia during atrial fibrillation with a rapid ventricular rate (this patient had not been treated with digoxin). The ECG in Figure 5.28 shows ischaemic ST segment depression in a patient with an AV nodal re-entry tachycardia and a ventricular rate of > 200/min.

Anterolateral ischaemia

Note
- Sinus rhythm
- Possible left atrial hypertrophy (bifid P wave in lead I)
- Normal axis
- Normal QRS complexes
- ST segment depression in leads I, II, V_4–V_6

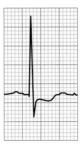

ST segment depression in lead V_5

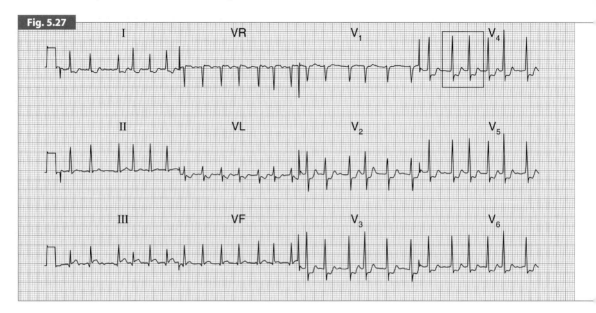

Fig. 5.27

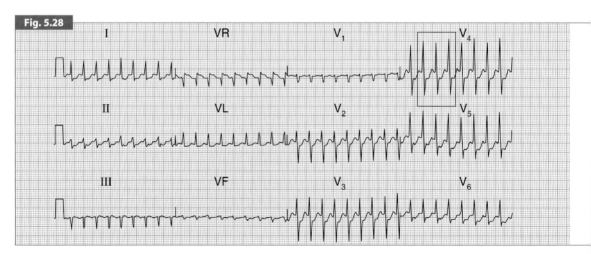

Fig. 5.28

Atrial fibrillation and anterior ischaemia

Note

- Atrial fibrillation, ventricular rate about 130/min
- Normal axis
- Normal QRS complexes
- ST segment depression in leads V_2–V_6

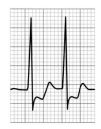

ST segment depression in lead V_4

AV nodal re-entry tachycardia with anterior ischaemia

Note

- Regular narrow complex tachycardia, rate 215/min
- No P waves
- ST segment depression in leads V_2–V_6

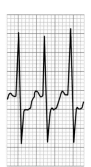

Narrow complexes and ST segment depression in lead V_4

245

Fig. 5.29

Prinzmetal's variant angina

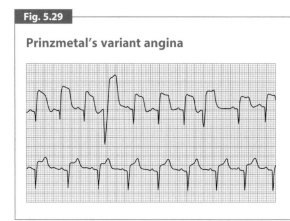

Note
- Continuous record
- Initially the patient had pain, and the ST segment was raised
- The fourth beat is probably a ventricular extrasystole
- As the patient's pain settled, the ST segment returned to normal

Fig. 5.30

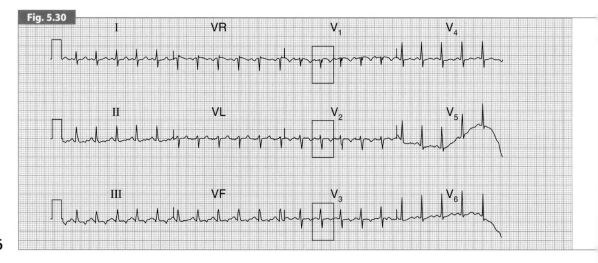

PRINZMETAL'S 'VARIANT' ANGINA

Angina can occur at rest due to spasm of the coronary arteries. This is accompanied by elevation rather than depression of the ST segments. The ECG appearance is similar to that of an acute myocardial infarction, but the ST segment returns to normal as the pain settles (Fig. 5.29). This ECG appearance was first described by Prinzmetal, and it is sometimes called 'variant' angina.

THE ECG IN PULMONARY EMBOLISM

Most patients with a pulmonary embolus will have sinus tachycardia, but an otherwise normal ECG.

The ECG abnormalities that may occur in pulmonary embolism are those associated with right ventricular problems:

- peaked P waves
- right axis deviation
- dominant R wave in lead V_1
- inverted T waves in leads V_1–V_3, and sometimes V_4
- right bundle branch block pattern
- shift in the transition point from leads V_3–V_4 to V_5–V_6, leading to a persistent deep S wave in lead V_6
- Q wave and inverted T wave in lead III.

Supraventricular arrhythmias, especially atrial fibrillation, may also occur. There is no particular sequence in which these changes develop, and they can be seen in any combination. The full ECG pattern of right ventricular hypertrophy (right axis deviation, dominant R waves in lead V_1, inverted T waves in leads V_1–V_4, and persistent S waves in lead V_6) is usually only seen in patients with long-standing thromboembolic pulmonary hypertension.

Figures 5.30, 5.31, 5.32 and 5.33 show the records from four patients with a pulmonary embolus – but remember, in most patients the ECG is normal.

Pulmonary embolus
Note
- Sinus rhythm, 130/min
- Normal axis
- Normal QRS complexes
- Inverted T wave in leads V_1–V_3, VF

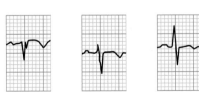

Inverted T wave in leads V_1–V_3

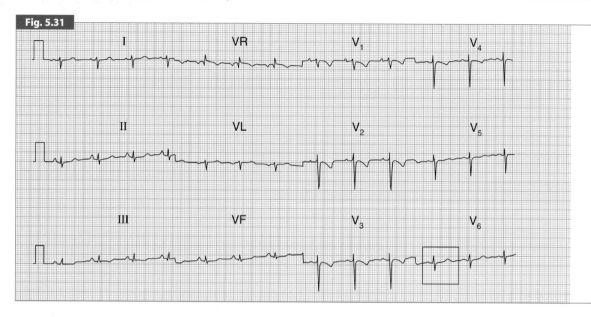

Fig. 5.31

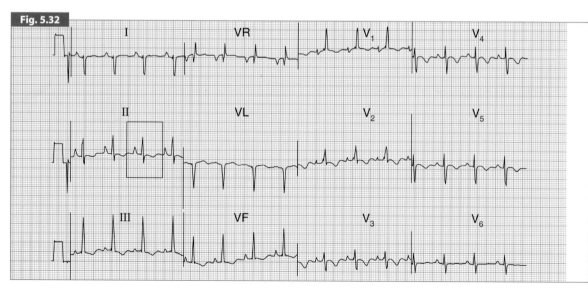

Fig. 5.32

Pulmonary embolus

Note
- Sinus rhythm
- Right axis deviation
- Persistent S wave in lead V_6
- T wave inversion in leads V_1–V_4

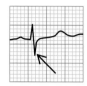

Persistent S wave in lead V_6

Pulmonary embolus

Note
- Sinus rhythm
- Peaked P wave suggests right atrial hypertrophy
- Right axis deviation
- Right bundle branch block pattern
- Persistent S wave in lead V_6
- T wave inversion in leads V_1–V_4

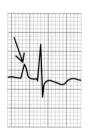

Peaked P wave in lead II

249

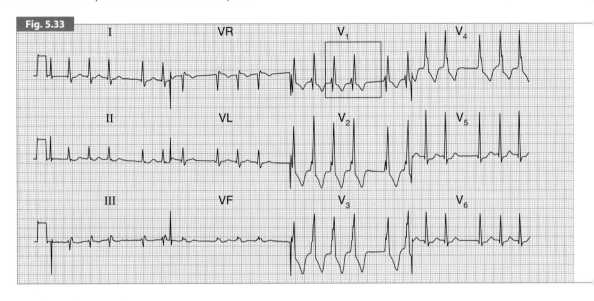

Fig. 5.33

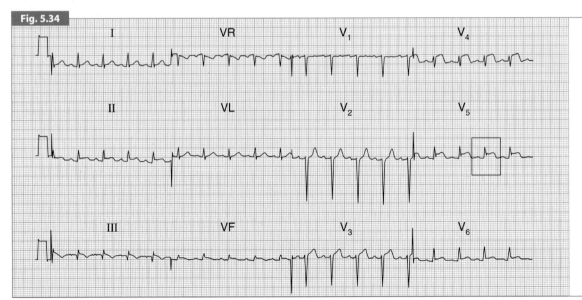

Fig. 5.34

Pulmonary embolus

Note

- Atrial fibrillation
- Right bundle branch block pattern

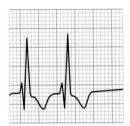

RSR¹ pattern in lead V₁

Pericarditis

Note

- Sinus rhythm
- Normal axis
- Normal QRS complexes
- ST segment elevation in leads I–III, VF, V₃–V₆

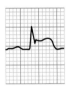

ST segment elevation in lead V₅

THE ECG IN OTHER CAUSES OF CHEST PAIN

PERICARDITIS

Pericarditis classically causes raised ST segments in most leads (Fig. 5.34). This may suggest a widespread acute infarction, but in pericarditis the ST segment remains elevated and Q waves do not develop. This pattern is actually very rare: most patients with pericarditis have either a normal ECG, or a variety of nonspecific ST segment/T wave changes.

AORTIC STENOSIS AND AORTIC DISSECTION

Aortic stenosis is an important cause of angina. The ECG should show left ventricular hypertrophy (Fig. 5.35). However, the ECG is an unreliable guide to left ventricular hypertrophy and the difficulty of distinguishing it from ischaemia is discussed in Chapter 6.

The presence of left ventricular hypertrophy in the ECG of a patient with chest pain also raises the possibility of aortic dissection.

Fig. 5.35

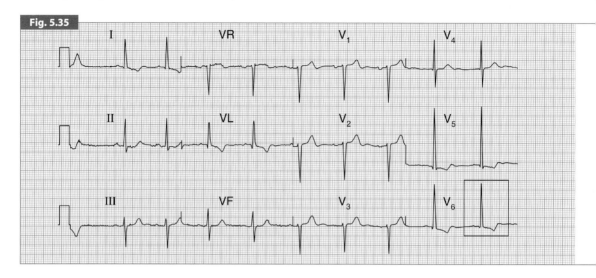

ECG PITFALLS IN THE DIAGNOSIS OF CHEST PAIN

The normal variants of the ECG have been described in Chapter 1. The important features that may cause confusion with ischaemia are:

- septal Q waves (mainly in leads II, VL, V_6)
- Q waves in lead III but not VF
- anterior T wave inversion (not uncommon in lead V_2, common in black people in leads V_2, V_3 and sometimes V_4)
- high take-off ST segments.

Several abnormal ECG patterns may cause difficulty in making a diagnosis in patients with chest pain, and some of these are summarized in Table 5.1. Other causes of 'false positives' include benign early repolarization (see Ch. 1), left bundle branch block, the Brugada syndrome, myocarditis and pericarditis, and pulmonary embolism. 'False negatives' may be the result of prior myocardial infarction with persistent ST segment elevation, a permanent pacemaker, or left bundle branch block. The conditions in which the ECG can give false positive or false negative results in the diagnosis of myocardial infarction are listed in Box 5.7.

Left ventricular hypertrophy

Note
- Sinus rhythm
- Tall R waves in leads V$_5$–V$_6$
- Inverted T waves in lateral leads

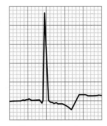

Tall R wave and inverted T wave in lead V$_6$

Table 5.1 **ECG pitfalls in the diagnosis of chest pain**

Condition	ECG pattern	May be confused with
Normal record	Q waves in lead III but not VF T wave inversion in leads V$_1$–V$_3$ (especially in black people)	Inferior infarction Anterior infarction
Left ventricular hypertrophy	T wave inversion in lateral leads	Ischaemia
Right ventricular hypertrophy	Dominant R waves in lead V$_1$ Inverted T waves in leads V$_1$–V$_3$	Posterior infarction Anterior infarction
The Wolff–Parkinson–White syndrome	Inverted T waves in leads V$_2$–V$_5$	Anterior infarction
Hypertrophic cardiomyopathy	T wave inversion in leads V$_2$–V$_5$	Anterior infarction
Subarachnoid haemorrhage	T wave inversion in any leads	Ischaemia
Digoxin effect	Downward-sloping ST segment depression or T wave inversion, especially in leads V$_5$–V$_6$	Ischaemia

Box 5.7 ECG pitfalls in diagnosing myocardial infarction

False positives
- Early repolarization
- Left bundle branch block
- Pre-excitation
- J point elevation syndromes, e.g. Brugada syndrome
- Pericarditis, myocarditis
- Pulmonary embolism
- Subarachnoid haemorrhage
- Metabolic disturbances, e.g. hyperkalaemia
- Cardiomyopathy
- Lead transposition

- Cholecystitis
- Malposition of precordial ECG electrodes
- Tricyclic antidepressants or phenothiazines

False negatives
- Prior myocardial infarction with Q waves and/or persistent ST segment elevation
- Right ventricular pacing
- Left bundle branch block

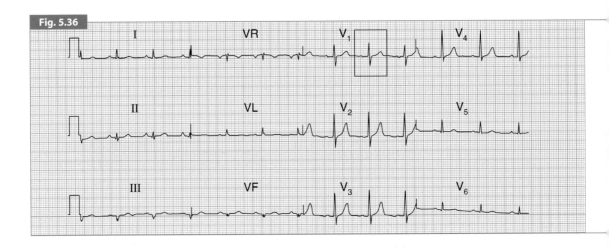

Fig. 5.36

R WAVE CHANGES

The ECG in Figure 5.36 shows a dominant R wave in lead V_1. This might be due to right ventricular hypertrophy or to a posterior infarction. Occasionally it could be a normal variant. Here, the normal axis goes against a diagnosis of right ventricular hypertrophy, and a review of previous ECGs from the patient showed that the dominant R wave was due to a posterior infarction.

The ECG in Figure 5.37 also shows a dominant R wave in lead V_1. In a patient with chest pain, a posterior infarction might again be considered. However, the PR interval is short and there is a delta wave, so this shows the Wolff–Parkinson–White (WPW) syndrome.

Old posterior infarction

Note
- Sinus rhythm
- Normal axis
- Dominant R waves in leads V_1–V_2
- No other abnormalities

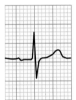

Dominant R wave in lead V_1

Fig. 5.37

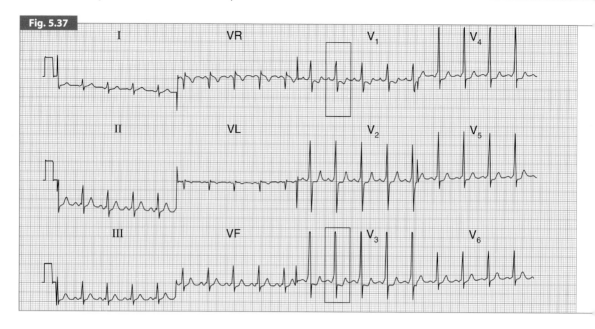

ST SEGMENT AND T WAVE CHANGES

It is, however, repolarization (T wave) changes that cause most problems. The lateral T wave inversion in the ECG in Figure 5.38 might suggest ischaemia, but again this is the WPW syndrome, in which repolarization abnormalities are common.

The anterior and lateral T wave inversion in the ECG in Figure 5.39 suggests either an NSTEMI or hypertrophic cardiomyopathy. This particular patient was white and asymptomatic, and had no family history of arrhythmias or any cardiac disease. There

was no echocardiographic evidence of cardiomyopathy, and coronary angiography was normal. The ECG reverted to normal on exercise, and the T wave inversion and the long QT interval remained unexplained.

Differentiation between lateral ischaemia and left ventricular hypertrophy on the ECG is extremely difficult. The ECG in Figure 5.40 shows lateral T wave inversion. There are small Q waves in leads III and VF, suggesting a possible old inferior infarction, and the QRS complexes in the chest leads are not particularly tall. Nevertheless, in this patient the lateral T wave inversion was due to left ventricular hypertrophy.

The Wolff–Parkinson–White syndrome type A

Note
- Sinus rhythm
- Short PR interval
- Slurred upstroke to QRS complexes
- Dominant R wave in lead V_1: the WPW syndrome type A

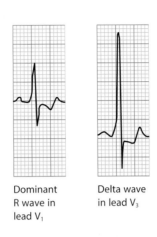

Dominant
R wave in
lead V_1

Delta wave
in lead V_3

The patient whose ECG is shown in Figure 5.41 had mild hypertension. The QRS complexes are tall (see Ch. 6) and there is lateral T wave inversion, suggesting left ventricular hypertrophy. However, there is also T wave inversion in leads V_3 and V_4, which is unusual in left ventricular hypertrophy. This patient had severe narrowing of the left main coronary artery.

Digoxin therapy causes downward-sloping ST segment depression and T wave inversion (see Ch. 7), particularly in the lateral leads, as is seen in Figure 5.42. The fact that the rhythm is atrial fibrillation with a controlled ventricular rate suggests that the patient is being treated with digoxin. However, T wave inversion in leads V_3 and V_4 is much more likely to be due to ischaemia, as was the case here.

An extremely common finding on the ECG is 'nonspecific T wave flattening' (Fig. 5.43). When a patient is completely well and the heart is clinically normal, this is of no importance. However, in a patient with chest pain that appears to be cardiac, 'nonspecific' ST segment/T wave changes may indicate ischaemia.

257

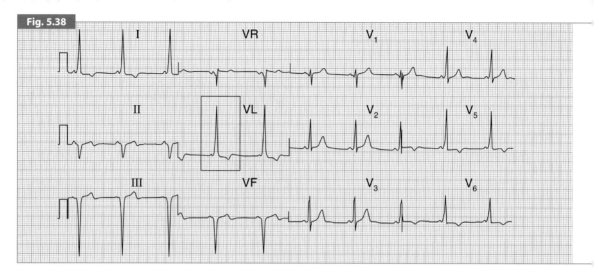

Fig. 5.38

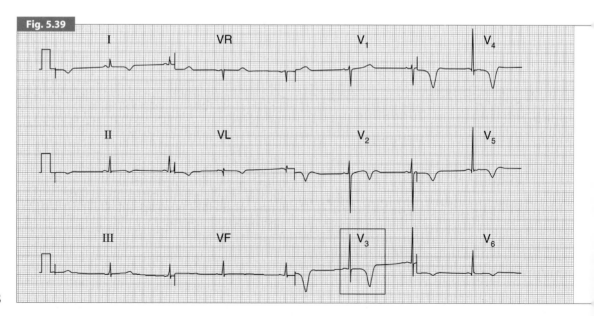

Fig. 5.39

The Wolff–Parkinson–White syndrome type B
Note
- Sinus rhythm
- Short PR interval
- Left axis deviation
- Delta wave
- Inverted T waves in leads I, VL, V_5–V_6
- No dominant R wave in lead V_1 (the WPW syndrome type B)

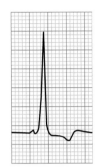

Short PR interval and delta wave in lead VL

Unexplained T wave abnormality
Note
- Sinus rhythm
- Normal axis
- Normal QRS complexes
- QT interval 600 ms
- T wave inversion in leads I–II, VL, V_2–V_6

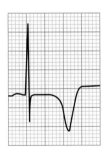

Long QT interval and inverted T wave in lead V_3

259

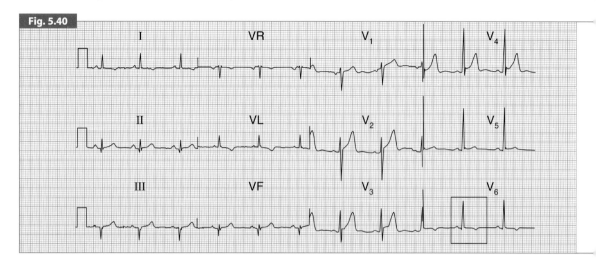

Fig. 5.40

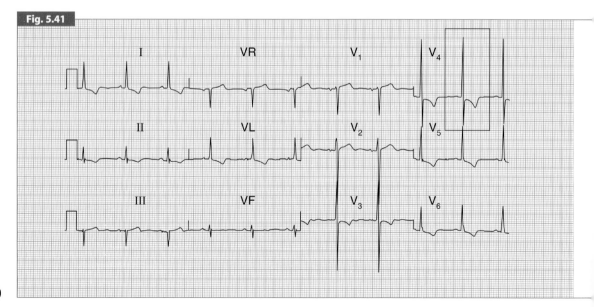

Fig. 5.41

Left ventricular hypertrophy
Note
- Sinus rhythm
- Normal axis
- Height of R wave in lead V_5 + depth of S wave in lead V_2 = 37 mm
- High take-off ST segment in lead V_4
- T wave inversion in leads I, VL, V_6

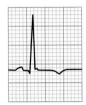

Inverted T wave in lead V_6

Old anterolateral NSTEMI
Note
- Sinus rhythm
- Normal axis
- Tall QRS complexes
- T wave inversion in leads I, VL, V_3–V_6, but this is more marked in lead V_4 than in V_6

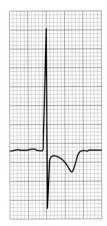

Inverted T wave in lead V_4

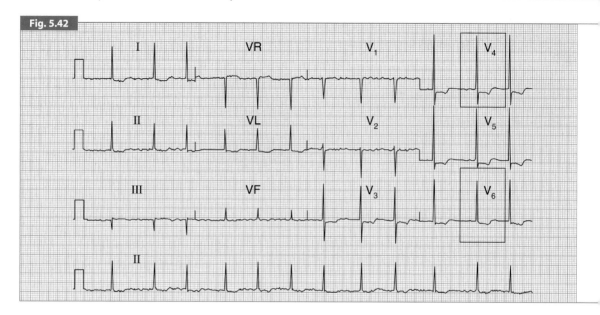

Fig. 5.42

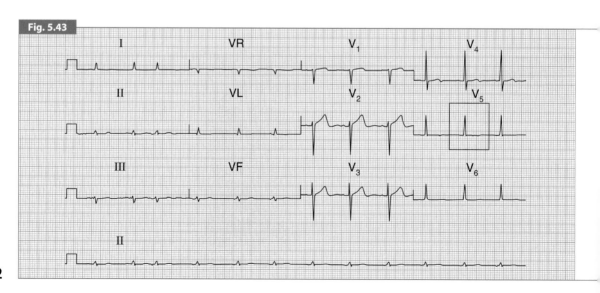

Fig. 5.43

Digoxin effect and ischaemia

Note

- Atrial fibrillation
- Normal axis
- Normal QRS complexes
- Horizontal ST segment depression in lead V_4
- Downward-sloping ST segment in lead V_6
- Inverted T waves in leads V_3–V_4

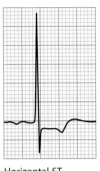

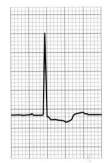

Horizontal ST
segment in lead V_4

Downward-sloping ST
segment in lead V_6

Nonspecific T wave flattening

Note

- Recorded at half sensitivity
- Sinus rhythm with supraventricular extrasystoles
- Normal QRS complexes
- Flat T waves in leads I, VL, V_5–V_6

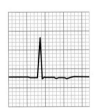

Flat T wave in lead V_5

WHAT TO DO ▶

It is essential to remember that while the ECG can on occasions be extremely helpful in the diagnosis of chest pain, frequently it is not. The history, and to a lesser extent the physical examination, are far more important. Serial changes in the ECG are more important than single records.

ACUTE CHEST PAIN SUGGESTING MYOCARDIAL INFARCTION

The treatment of patients with chest pain differs, depending on whether the ECG shows ST segment elevation (STEMI) or not (NSTEMI). Both patient categories can be said to have an 'acute coronary syndrome', though this is often used as if it were synonymous with NSTEMI.

The ECG can be normal in the first few hours of the onset of a STEMI, so in order to differentiate between a STEMI and an NSTEMI it is essential that 12-lead ECGs should be repeated at least hourly until the diagnosis is clear. Blood samples should be taken immediately to identify troponin (T or I) and CK-MB levels. However, it is important to remember that the plasma troponin levels may not rise for up to 12 h, so the test should not be considered negative until 12 h after the onset of chest pain.

OTHER INVESTIGATIONS FOR PATIENTS WITH ACUTE CHEST PAIN

Chest X-rays are seldom helpful. Unless a pneumothorax or some other cause of pleurisy, or a dissecting aneurysm, seems possible the patient should not be detained waiting for an X-ray examination. Chest X-rays taken using portable equipment are rarely useful.

Echocardiography is the investigation of choice if pericarditis is suspected, because most patients will have a pericardial effusion which is easily detected. Subsequent treatment will depend on the underlying cause of the pericarditis. Possible causes are listed in Box 5.8.

Box 5.8 Causes of pericarditis

- Viruses
- Bacteria (including tuberculosis)
- Dressler's syndrome after myocardial infarction
- Malignancy
- Uraemia
- Acute rheumatic fever
- Myxoedema
- Connective tissue disease
- Radiotherapy

Echocardiography may also help in the diagnosis of an aortic dissection, but not reliably – CT scanning is probably the investigation of choice in such cases. Echocardiography may also be helpful in suspected pulmonary embolism, because it may show right ventricular dilatation.

THE INVESTIGATION OF CHRONIC CHEST PAIN

Chronic or intermittent chest pain must be investigated and treated as the history dictates. Chronic chest pain that could be due to coronary disease is very common, and there is a long list of possible investigations, with varying accuracy of diagnosis, risk or discomfort for the patient, and cost. The 'gold standard' investigation might seem to be coronary angiography, but anatomical coronary disease is not necessarily the cause of a patient's symptoms. There is no single test that fulfils all the criteria of high sensitivity and specificity, absence of risk and discomfort, and low cost.

Clinical guidelines issued by the National Institute of Health and Clinical Excellence suggest that the key to the diagnosis of angina is the clinical assessment (NICE clinical guideline 95: *Chest pain of recent onset: assessment and diagnosis of recent onset chest pain or discomfort of suspected cardiac origin* (2010)). Anginal pain is constricting, and radiates to the neck, jaw or arms; it is precipitated by physical exertion and it is rapidly relieved by rest or glyceryl trinitrate. The guidelines suggest that if only some of these features are present, the term 'atypical angina' should be used. The guidelines also suggest that if only one feature is present, the pain should be defined as 'non-anginal'. A patient can be considered to be at high risk of having coronary artery disease (CAD) if they have diabetes and hyperlipidaemia, and are a smoker.

The percentage of people estimated to have CAD according to their age, gender, symptoms and risk factors is shown in Table 5.2.

The two essential investigations in a patient with stable and chronic chest pain are the ECG and the measurement of blood haemoglobin, to identify conditions that exacerbate angina, such as anaemia. After these, NICE guidelines suggest that if the estimated likelihood of CAD is greater than 90%, no further diagnostic tests are needed. If the likelihood of CAD is less than 10%, investigation should be aimed at causes of chest pain other than angina; or, if the symptoms are typical of angina, at causes of angina other than CAD, such as hypertrophic cardiomyopathy or aortic stenosis.

Table 5.2 Percentage of people estimated to have coronary artery disease

Age (years)	Non-anginal chest pain		Atypical angina		Typical angina	
	Low risk	High risk	Low risk	High risk	Low risk	High risk
Men						
35	3	35	8	59	30	88
55	23	59	45	79	80	95
65	49	69	71	86	93	97
>70			>90	>90	>90	>90
Women						
35	1	19	2	39	10	78
55	4	25	10	47	38	82
65	9	29	20	51	56	84
>70	61–90	61–90	61–90	61–90	61–90	>90

Values are per cent of people at each mid-decade age with significant coronary artery disease.
High risk = diabetes, smoking and hyperlipidaemia (total cholesterol > 6.47 mmol/litre).
Low risk = none of these three.

National Institute for Health and Clinical Excellence (2010). Adapted from CG 95 Chest pain of recent onset: assessment and diagnosis of recent onset chest pain or discomfort of suspected cardiac origin. London: NICE. Available from http://guidance.nice.org.uk/CG95. Reproduced with permission. Content accurate at time of going to press.

The NICE guidelines suggest that if the likelihood of CAD is 61–90%, the first-line diagnostic investigation is invasive coronary angiography, if clinically indicated. If the likelihood of CAD is 30–60%, some form of functional imaging should be used; and if the likelihood is 10–29%, the first-line diagnostic investigation should be CT calcium scoring. CT scoring has a higher diagnostic sensitivity than exercise testing, and so it is more useful as a first test for excluding coronary disease, and thus for avoiding a further sequence of tests. When considering the use of CT calcium scoring the risks of radiation (roughly equivalent to a barium swallow) must be taken into account.

The non-invasive functional imaging tests considered in the NICE guidelines include myocardial perfusion scintigraphy with single-photon emission computed tomography (MPS with SPECT), stress echocardiography, first-pass contrast-enhanced magnetic resonance (MR) perfusion, or MR imaging for stress-induced wall motion abnormalities. Features of these techniques, in order of common availability, are summarized in Table 5.3.

The exercise ECG is thus not regarded as a useful test for the diagnosis of angina, and the guidelines suggest that its remaining use is in the assessment of functional capacity in patients with known coronary artery disease. However, even though exercise testing is undoubtedly less sensitive and less specific than the other tests, it is still probably the most widely used investigation for chest pain, because of its advantages. Above all, it provides an opportunity to assess and judge the patient as a whole (Box 5.9) and to see what workload they can achieve, and whether the limiting factor is chest pain or some other factor, such as joint pain or anxiety.

Box 5.9 Information obtainable from exercise testing

- The patient's attitude to exercise
- The reasons for exercise limitation
  - chest pain
  - breathlessness
  - claudication
  - fatigue
  - musculoskeletal problems
- The pumping capability of the heart
  - maximum heart rate achieved
  - maximum rise in blood pressure
- Physical fitness
  - workload at which maximum heart rate is achieved
  - duration of tachycardia following exercise
- Ischaemic changes in the ECG
- Exercise-induced arrhythmias

Table 5.3 **Possible non-invasive investigations in chronic chest pain**

Investigation	Stressor	Sensitivity/specificity*
Exercise test	Exercise	Sensitivity ~68% Specificity ~77%
Stress echocardiography	Exercise Dobutamine Vasodilators (e.g. adenosine, dipyridamole)	Sensitivity ~79% Specificity ~87%
Myocardial perfusion scintigraphy	Exercise Dobutamine Vasodilators (e.g. adenosine, or dipyridamole used as a safe vasodilator)	Sensitivity ~88% Specificity ~73%
Stress MRI	Exercise (rare) Dobutamine Vasodilators (e.g. adenosine, dipyridamole)	Sensitivity ~91% Specificity ~81%
Cardiac CT scoring	None	CT calcium score 0: Sensitivity ~94% CT angiography: Sensitivity ~94% Specificity 88–97%

* Note sensitivity and specificity for all tests depend on the pre-test probability of coronary disease in the patient population studied. This should be considered when interpreting the results of any diagnostic test and when selecting the most appropriate test. Hence patients with higher pre-test probabilities will have higher false negative rates, and patients with lower pre-test probabilities will have higher false positive rates.

Advantages	Disadvantages
Widely available; low cost Safe (death/myocardial infarction 1:2500) Quick to perform Can be carried out by a trained technician Exercise capacity is a good indication of the patient's overall functional state and prognosis	Limited ability to localize coronary disease Difficult to interpret if ECG baseline abnormal (e.g. with left bundle branch block (LBBB), pacing, Wolff–Parkinson–White syndrome or left ventricular hypertrophy) Some patients are physically unable to perform adequately Less sensitive in women Reduced sensitivity and specificity compared with other tests
Single attendance (about 1 h) Can quantify and localize ischaemic and infarcted territory Not affected by baseline ECG or functional capacity, although may be harder to interpret with atrial fibrillation Can evaluate valves during the same investigation	Requires considerable operator expertise 5–10% inadequate echo windows Indirect assessment of perfusion Risk of ventricular tachycardia (VT) (1:1500 with dipyridamole, 1:300 with dobutamine) May be difficult to stress if paced or beta-blocked, or with LBBB
Can quantify and localize ischaemic and infarcted territory Not affected by baseline ECG, including atrial fibrillation or by patient's exercise capacity Direct assessment of perfusion	Longer attendance: often over 2 days Radiation dose (~6 mSv) Risk of VT (1:1500 with dipyridamole, 1:300 with dobutamine) May be difficult to stress if paced or beta-blocked, or with LBBB Requires considerable operator and reporter expertise Balanced defects in multivessel disease may lead to false negatives
High quality images, more consistent than with stress echocardiography Can assess perfusion, functional ischaemia and valves Single attendance (about 1 h)	Claustrophobia Difficult with atrial fibrillation Contraindicated with metallic implants, including pacemakers Risk of VT (1:1500 with dipyridamole, 1:300 with dobutamine) Requires considerable operator and reporter expertise
CT calcium score quick to perform and interpret (5 min) CT calcium score good screening tool, especially for patients with low pre-test probability Only non-invasive means to assess coronary anatomy	Radiation dose 1.5–3 mSv for CT calcium score, ~10 mSv for CT angiogram Patients with positive calcium scores will require further investigation with either CT angiography, functional assessment or coronary angiography An anatomical test, so no assessment of function

Table 5.4 Bruce protocol for exercise testing using a treadmill, 3 min at each stage

Stage	Speed		Slope		METS (metabolic equivalents)
	Miles per hour	Kilometres per hour	Grade (%)	Degrees to horizontal	
Low level					
01	1.7	2.7	0	0	2.9
02	1.7	2.7	5	2.9	3.7
Standard Bruce protocol					
1	1.7	2.7	10	5.7	5.0
2	2.5	4.0	12	6.8	7.0
3	3.4	5.5	14	8.0	9.5
4	4.2	6.8	16	9.1	13.5
5	5.0	8.0	18	10.2	17.0

EXERCISE TESTING

Although any form of exercise that induces pain should produce ischaemic changes in the ECG, it is best to use a reproducible test that patients find reasonably easy to perform, and to use carefully graded increments of exercise. The use of non-standard tests means that the results may be difficult to interpret, and that repeated tests in the same patient cannot be compared meaningfully.

PRACTICAL ASPECTS OF EXERCISE TESTING

Reproducible exercise testing needs either a bicycle ergometer or a treadmill. In either case, the exercise should begin at a low level that the patient finds easy, and should be made progressively more difficult. On a bicycle, the pedal speed should be kept constant and the workload increased in steps of 25 watts. On a treadmill, both the slope and the speed can be changed

and the protocol evolved by Bruce (Table 5.4) is the one most commonly used.

The workload achieved by a patient on a treadmill is sometimes expressed as metabolic equivalents (METS). The rate at which oxygen is used by an average person at rest is 1 MET, and it equals 3.5 ml/kg/min. However, few people are average, and oxygen consumption is dependent on weight, age and gender, so METS are not particularly useful. Box 5.10

Box 5.10 Average workloads, expressed in metabolic equivalents

Activity	METS
Cleaning floors	4.0
Gardening	4.0
Sexual intercourse	5.0
Bed making	5.0–6.0
Carrying a medium suitcase	7.0

shows the estimated workloads imposed by various activities, and hence how exercise tolerance (as measured on the treadmill) indicates what a patient might be expected to achieve.

A 12-lead ECG, the heart rate and the blood pressure should be recorded at the end of each exercise period. The maximum heart rate and blood pressure are in some ways more important than the maximum workload achieved, because the latter is markedly influenced by physical fitness. However, the ECG recorded during exercise testing is unreliable in cases of:

- bundle branch block
- ventricular hypertrophy
- the Wolff–Parkinson–White syndrome
- digoxin therapy
- beta-blocker therapy.

REASONS FOR DISCONTINUING AN EXERCISE TEST

1. At the request of the patient – because of pain, breathlessness, fatigue or dizziness.
2. If the systolic blood pressure begins to fall. Normally, systolic pressure will rise progressively with increasing exercise level, but in any subject a point will be reached at which systolic pressure reaches a plateau and then starts to fall. A fall of 10 mmHg is an indication that the heart is not pumping effectively and the test should be stopped – if it is continued, the patient will become dizzy and may fall. In healthy subjects, a fall in systolic pressure is seen only at high workloads, but in patients with severe heart disease the systolic pressure may fail to rise on exercise. The amount of exercise the patient can carry out before the systolic pressure falls is thus a useful indicator of the severity of any heart disease.

3. It is conventional to discontinue the test if the heart rate increases to 80% of the predicted maximum for the patient's age. This maximum can be calculated in beats/min by subtracting the patient's age in years from 220. Patients with severe heart disease will usually fail to attain 80% of their predicted maximum heart rate, and the peak rate is another useful indicator of the state of the patient's heart. It is, of course, important to take note of any treatment the patient may be receiving, because a beta-blocker will prevent the normal increase in heart rate.
4. Exercise should be discontinued immediately if an arrhythmia occurs. Many patients will have ventricular extrasystoles during exercise. These can be ignored unless their frequency begins to rise, or a couplet of extrasystoles occurs.
5. The test should be stopped if the ST segment in any lead becomes depressed by 4 mm. Horizontal depression of 2 mm in any lead is usually taken as indicating that a diagnosis of ischaemia can be made (a 'positive' test), and if the aim of the test is to confirm or refute a diagnosis of angina there is no point in continuing once this has occurred. It may, however, be useful to find out just how much a patient can do, and if this is the aim of the test it is not unreasonable to continue, if the patient's symptoms are not severe.

INTERPRETATION OF ECG CHANGES DURING EXERCISE TESTING

The final report of the test should indicate the duration of exercise, the workload achieved, the maximum heart rate and systolic pressure, the reason for discontinuing the test, and a description of any arrhythmias or ST segment changes.

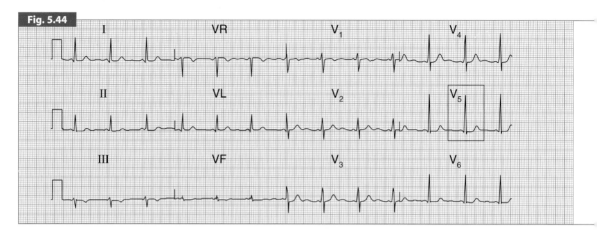

Fig. 5.44

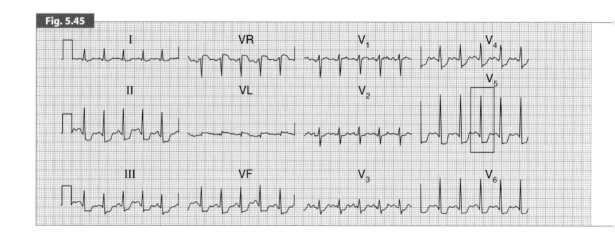

Fig. 5.45

Probably normal record

Note
- Sinus rhythm
- Normal axis
- Normal QRS complexes
- Some nonspecific T wave change in leads III, VF

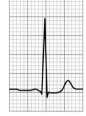

Normal ST segment in lead V₅

Exercise-induced ischaemia

Note
- Same patient as in Figure 5.44
- Sinus rhythm, 138/min
- Horizontal ST segment depression in leads II–III, VF, V₄–V₆

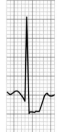

Horizontal ST segment depression in lead V₅

An exercise test is usually considered 'positive' for ischaemia if horizontal or downward-sloping ST segment depression of 2 mm or more develops during exercise, and resolves on resting. By convention, ST segment depression is measured relative to the ECG baseline (between the T and P waves) 60–80 ms after the J point (the point of inflection at the junction of the S wave and the ST segment). A diagnosis of ischaemia becomes almost certain if these changes are accompanied by the appearance and then disappearance of angina. Figures 5.44 and 5.45 show an ECG that was normal when the patient was at rest, but which demonstrated clear ischaemia during exercise. Box 5.11 lists the normal changes in the ECG during exercise, and Box 5.12 lists the changes suggesting a high probability of coronary disease.

Box 5.11 Normal ECG changes during exercise

- P wave increases in height
- R wave decreases in height
- J point becomes depressed
- ST segment becomes upward-sloping
- QT interval shortens
- T wave decreases in height

Box 5.12 Changes on exercise suggesting a high probability of coronary artery disease

ECG changes
- Horizontal ST segment depression of > 2 mm
- Downward-sloping ST segment depression
- Positive response (i.e. ST segment changes) within 6 min
- Persistence of ST segment depression for more than 6 min into recovery
- ST segment depression in five or more leads

Other changes
- Exertional hypotension

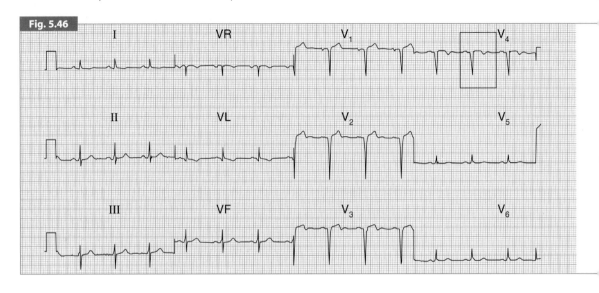

Fig. 5.46

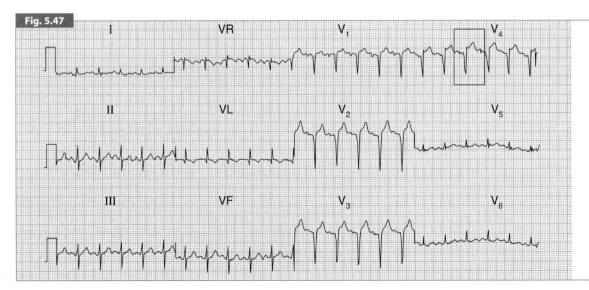

Fig. 5.47

Anterior infarction, ?age

Note
- Sinus rhythm
- Normal axis
- Q waves in leads V_2–V_4
- Slight ST segment elevation in leads V_2–V_4

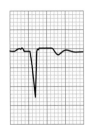

Q wave, slight ST segment elevation and
inverted T wave in lead V_4

Exercise-induced ST segment elevation

Note
- Same patient as in Figure 5.46
- The ST segments are now higher in leads V_3–V_4

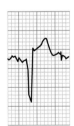

More ST segment elevation
in lead V_4

There are, however, other ECG changes that may be seen during an exercise test. Figures 5.46 and 5.47 show the records of tests in a patient who had had an anterior myocardial infarction some weeks previously. At rest, some ST segment elevation persisted in the anterior leads. During exercise the ST elevation became more marked. The reasons for this are uncertain. It has been suggested that the change is due to the development of an abnormality of left ventricular contraction, but other evidence suggests that it is simply another ECG manifestation of ischaemia. There is, however, no doubt that this is an abnormal result.

When the resting ECG shows T wave inversion and on exercise the T waves become upright, this is called 'pseudonormalization', and it is a sign of ischaemia (Fig. 5.48).

Fig. 5.48

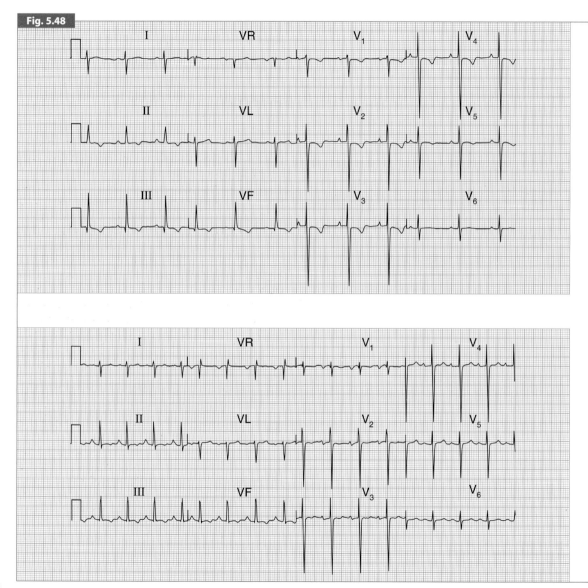

Pseudonormalization

Note

At rest (upper trace):

- Right axis deviation
- Small Q waves with inverted T waves in leads III and VF suggest an old inferior infarction
- T wave inversion in leads II and V_2–V_4 suggests ischaemia (T wave inversion in lead V_1 is normal)

On exercise (lower trace):

- Q waves disappear
- T wave inversion partly 'normalizes' in lead II and completely 'normalizes' in the chest leads, but persists in lead VF

This pattern suggests the pseudonormalization of an ECG showing ischaemia at rest

When the J point and the ST segment become depressed during exercise, but the ST segment slopes upwards, the change is not an indication of ischaemia (Figs 5.49 and 5.50). Deciding whether ST segment depression slopes upwards or is horizontal can be quite difficult.

False positive changes also occur when exercise testing is performed in patients taking digoxin. Figures 5.51 and 5.52 show the results of an exercise test in a patient being treated with digoxin, whose coronary angiogram was normal.

In a patient suspected of having coronary disease, exercise testing gives the 'right' answer in about 75% of patients tested – to be more precise, exercise testing has a sensitivity of 68% and a specificity of 77%. All tests at times give false positive and false negative results, reflecting their specificity and sensitivity, and false positive tests are particularly common in middle-aged women. In an asymptomatic subject in whom the likelihood of coronary disease is low, the chance of a false positive result may be higher than the chance of a true positive. Also, the greater the likelihood that the patient has coronary disease, the more likely it is that a positive test is 'true' rather than 'false'. The statistics (Bayes' theorem) may seem complex, but the important thing is to remember that exercise testing is not infallible.

Some patients who give a history characteristic of angina, and who have an undoubtedly positive exercise test according to their ECG, have normal coronary arteries. This condition is called 'Cardiac Syndrome X'. In some cases the patient has structural heart disease (e.g. left ventricular hypertrophy, mitral valve prolapse, myocardial bridging), but most patients have an apparently normal heart and the cause of Cardiac Syndrome X is unknown.

Exercise testing thus has to be used and interpreted with care.

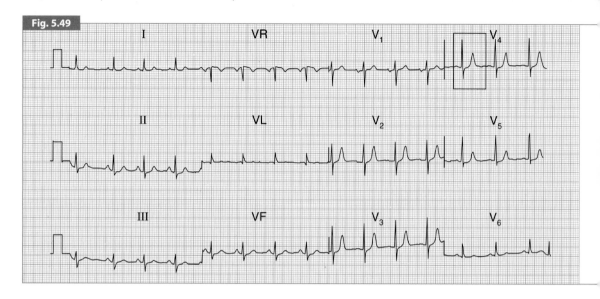

Fig. 5.49

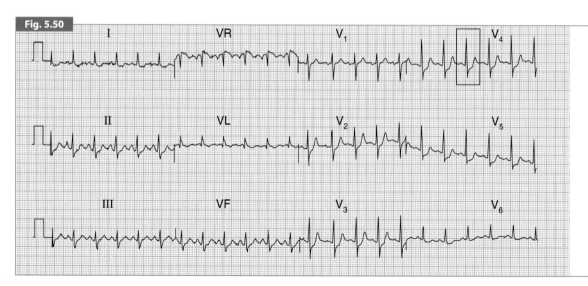

Fig. 5.50

Normal ECG
Note
- Sinus rhythm
- Normal axis
- Normal QRS complexes
- Possible minimal ST segment depression in lead V_5

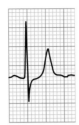

Normal ST segment in lead V_4

Exercise-induced ST segment depression
Note
- Same patient as Figure 5.49
- On exercise there is ST segment depression which slopes upwards
- This is not diagnostic of ischaemia, but the change in lead V_5 is suspicious

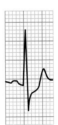

Upward-sloping ST segment depression in lead V_4

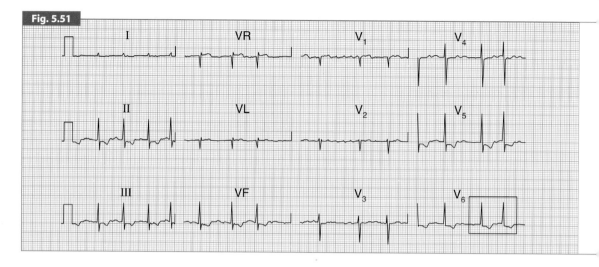

Fig. 5.51

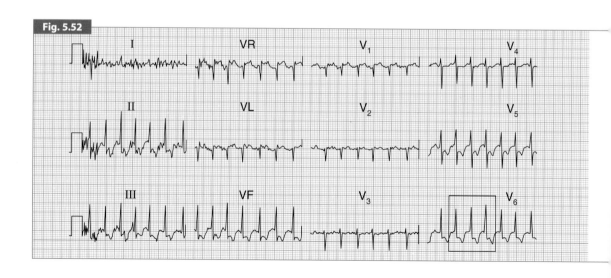

Fig. 5.52

Atrial fibrillation: digoxin effect at rest

Note
- Atrial fibrillation
- ST segments slope downwards and T waves are inverted in leads V₅–V₆: typical of digoxin effect

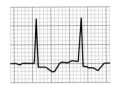

Downward-sloping ST segment and inverted T wave in lead V₆

Atrial fibrillation: digoxin effect on exercise

Note
- Same patient as Figure 5.51
- Heart rate 165/min
- ST segment depression in lead V₆ could be ischaemic but could be a false positive due to digoxin

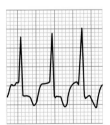

Further ST segment depression in lead V₆

RISKS OF EXERCISE TESTING

Exercise testing involves a risk of about 1 in 5000 of the development of ventricular tachycardia or ventricular fibrillation, and a risk of about 1 in 10000 tests of myocardial infarction or death. There is also a risk of injury if the patient falls, or jumps, off the treadmill. Box 5.13 lists some contraindications of exercise testing.

The ECGs in Figures 5.53, 5.54 and 5.55 are from a patient whose resting ECG was normal, but as the test proceeded he began to develop ventricular extrasystoles and then suddenly developed ventricular fibrillation. This demonstrates the need for full resuscitation facilities to be available at the time of exercise testing.

Fig. 5.53

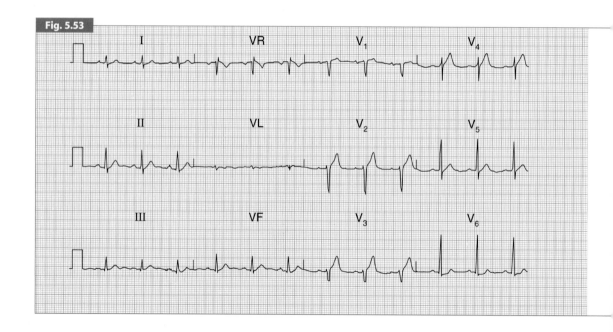

Box 5.13 **Contraindications of exercise testing**

- Acute myocardial infarction within preceding 4–6 days
- Unstable angina
- Uncontrolled heart failure
- Acute myocarditis or pericarditis
- Deep vein thrombosis
- Uncontrolled hypertension (systolic > 220 mmHg, diastolic > 120 mmHg
- Severe aortic stenosis
- Severe hypertrophic cardiomyopathy
- Untreated life-threatening arrhythmia

Pre-exercise: normal ECG

Note

- Sinus rhythm
- Heart rate 75/min
- Possible nonspecific ST segment depression in lead V_6

Fig. 5.54

Exercise-induced ventricular extrasystoles

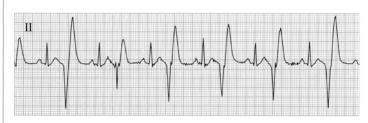

Note
- Same patient as in Figure 5.53
- Sinus rhythm with coupled ventricular extrasystoles

Fig. 5.55

Exercise-induced ventricular fibrillation

Note
- Same patient as in Figures 5.53 and 5.54
- One sinus beat is followed by an extrasystole with the R on T phenomenon
- A few beats of ventricular tachycardia decay into ventricular fibrillation

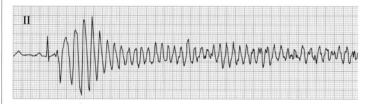

MANAGEMENT OF CHEST PAIN

STEMI

Patients with STEMI require immediate coronary recanalization by means of either percutaneous coronary intervention (PCI) or thrombolysis.

NSTEMI

Patients with NSTEMI should be treated immediately with aspirin, low-molecular-weight heparin, clopidogrel, a beta-blocker (provided there are no contraindications), a statin and nitrates.

Two risk categories of NSTEMI can be identified, which require different subsequent treatments.

Patients at high risk have any of:

- persistent or recurrent chest pain
- ST segment depression
- diabetes
- elevated troponin levels
- haemodynamic instability
- rhythm instability.

In addition to the baseline treatment above, these patients require an infusion of a glycoprotein IIb/IIIa inhibitor followed by coronary angiography before discharge from hospital. Angiography is urgent in unstable patients. Most high-risk patients will need angioplasty or bypass surgery, often as a matter of urgency.

Low-risk patients include those with all of:

- no recurrent chest pain
- an ECG showing T wave inversion, flat T waves or no ECG changes at all
- normal troponin levels after 12 h.

Heparin can be discontinued but aspirin, beta-blockers, nitrates, a statin and clopidogrel are continued. As soon as possible, an exercise or another non-invasive test should be performed to assess the probability and severity of coronary disease. On the basis of the test results and the clinical picture, a decision can be made about the need for, and urgency of, coronary angiography.

LONG-TERM TREATMENT AFTER MYOCARDIAL INFARCTION

In all patients it is important to manage risk factors aggressively, with the cessation of smoking, weight control and regular exercise. Aspirin, beta-blockers and statins are needed indefinitely, and clopidogrel for 9 months.

CHRONIC CHEST PAIN

A trial of sublingual glyceryl trinitrate 0.5 mg may help make the diagnosis of angina, and in such cases patients should then be encouraged to use the drug liberally and prophylactically. Beta-blockers are the first-line agents for preventing angina. If the patient is unable to take a beta-blocker (e.g. because of asthma), treatment should start with a calcium-channel blocker such as amlodipine. Nicorandil and ivabradine may also be useful, especially in patients intolerant of other drugs. All these drugs can be combined, or a long-acting nitrate such as isosorbide mononitrate can be substituted for one of these classes of drug. A combination of two of these drug classes is sometimes helpful; the addition of the third seldom provides much further benefit. Secondary prophylactic measures, including aspirin and a statin, are essential.

Otherwise, treatment will depend on the cause of the chest pain. If investigation (see above) reveals that the cause is cardiac, and despite maximum medical therapy the patient remains symptomatic, invasive procedures such as coronary artery bypass grafting or percutaneous transluminal coronary angioplasty may need to be considered.

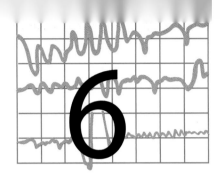

The ECG in patients with breathlessness

History and examination	287
Rhythm problems	291
The ECG in disorders affecting the left side of the heart	293
The ECG in left atrial hypertrophy	293
The ECG in left ventricular hypertrophy	295
ECGs that can mimic left ventricular hypertrophy	299
The ECG in disorders affecting the right side of the heart	303
The ECG in right atrial hypertrophy	305
The ECG in right ventricular hypertrophy	305
What to do	312
Cardiac resynchronization therapy (CRT)	312

HISTORY AND EXAMINATION

There are many causes of breathlessness (see Box 6.1). Everyone is breathless at times, but people who are physically unfit or who are overweight will be more breathless than others. Breathlessness can also result from anxiety, but when it is due to physical illness the important causes are anaemia, heart disease and lung disease; a combination of causes is common. Apart from ischaemia (see Ch. 5), cardiac diseases causing breathlessness include valve disease, cardiomyopathy, and myocarditis including acute rheumatic fever. Boxes 6.2–6.6 summarize the effects of these conditions on the heart, and the corresponding ECG features. The most important function of the history is to help to determine whether the patient does indeed have a physical illness and, if so, which system is affected.

Breathlessness in heart disease is due to either increased lung stiffness, as a result of pulmonary congestion, or pulmonary oedema. Pulmonary congestion occurs when the left atrial pressure is high. A high left

Box 6.1 Underlying causes of breathlessness

Physiological and psychological
- Lack of fitness
- Obesity
- Pregnancy
- Locomotor diseases (including ankylosing spondylitis and neurological diseases)
- Anxiety

Heart disease – left ventricular failure
- Ischaemia
- Mitral regurgitation
- Aortic stenosis
- Aortic regurgitation
- Congenital disease
- Cardiomyopathy
- Myocarditis
- Arrhythmias

Heart disease – high left atrial pressure
- Mitral stenosis
- Atrial myxoma

Lung disease
- Chronic obstructive pulmonary disease
- Any interstitial lung disease (e.g. infection, tumour, infiltration)
- Pulmonary embolism
- Pleural effusion
- Pneumothorax

Pericardial disease
- Constrictive pericarditis

Anaemia

Box 6.2 The ECG in valve disease

Mitral stenosis
- Atrial fibrillation
- Left atrial hypertrophy, if in sinus rhythm
- Right ventricular hypertrophy

Mitral regurgitation
- Atrial fibrillation
- Left atrial hypertrophy, if in sinus rhythm
- Left ventricular hypertrophy

Aortic stenosis
- Left ventricular hypertrophy
- Incomplete left bundle branch block (i.e. loss of Q waves in leads V_5–V_6)
- Left bundle branch block

Aortic regurgitation
- Left ventricular hypertrophy
- Prominent but narrow Q wave in lead V_6
- Left anterior hemiblock
- Occasionally, left bundle branch block

Mitral valve prolapse
- Sinus rhythm, or wide variety of arrhythmias
- Inverted T waves in leads II–III, VF
- T wave inversion in precordial leads
- ST segment depression
- Exercise-induced ventricular arrhythmias

Note: abnormalities can vary in different records from the same individual

Biventricular hypertrophy
- Left ventricular hypertrophy plus right axis deviation
- Left ventricular hypertrophy plus clockwise rotation
- Left ventricular hypertrophy with tall R waves in lead V_1

Box 6.3 The ECG in congestive cardiomyopathy

- Arrhythmias, especially atrial fibrillation and ventricular tachycardia
- First degree block
- Right or left atrial enlargement
- Low amplitude QRS complexes
- Left anterior hemiblock
- Left bundle branch block
- Right bundle branch block
- Left ventricular hypertrophy
- Nonspecific ST segment and T wave changes

Box 6.4 The ECG in hypertrophic cardiomyopathy

- Short PR interval
- Various rhythm disturbances, including ventricular tachycardia and ventricular fibrillation
- Left atrial hypertrophy
- Left anterior hemiblock or left bundle branch block
- Left ventricular hypertrophy
- Prolonged QT interval
- Deep T wave inversion in the anterior leads

Box 6.5 The ECG in myocarditis

- Sinus tachycardias and other arrhythmias
- First, second or third degree block
- Widened QRS complexes
- Irregularity of QRS waveform
- Q waves
- Prolonged QT interval
- ST segment elevation or depression
- T wave inversion in any lead

Box 6.6 The ECG in acute rheumatic fever

- Sinus tachycardia
- First degree block
- ST segment/T wave changes of acute myocarditis
- Changes associated with pericarditis

atrial pressure occurs either in mitral stenosis or in left ventricular failure. Pulmonary oedema occurs when the left atrial pressure exceeds the oncotic pressure exerted by the plasma proteins.

Congestive cardiac failure (right heart failure secondary to left heart failure) can be difficult to distinguish from cor pulmonale (right heart failure due to lung disease). With both, the patient is breathless. Both are associated with pulmonary crackles – in left heart failure due to pulmonary oedema, and in cor pulmonale due to the lung disease. Also in both, the patient may complain of orthopnoea. In heart failure, this is due to the return to the effective circulation of blood that was pooled in the legs. In patients with chest disease (especially chronic obstructive airways disease), orthopnoea results from the need to use diaphragmatic respiration. Both pulmonary congestion and lung disease can cause a diffuse wheeze. The diagnosis therefore depends on a positive identification, either in the history or on examination, of heart or lung disease.

The main value of the ECG in patients with breathlessness is to indicate whether heart disease of any sort is present, and whether the left or the right side of the heart is affected. The ECG is best at identifying rhythm abnormalities (which may lead to left ventricular impairment and so to breathlessness) and conditions affecting the left ventricle – particularly ischaemia. The patient with a completely normal ECG is unlikely to have left ventricular failure, though of course there are exceptions. Lung disease eventually affects the right side of the heart, and may cause ECG changes suggesting that significant lung disease is present.

289

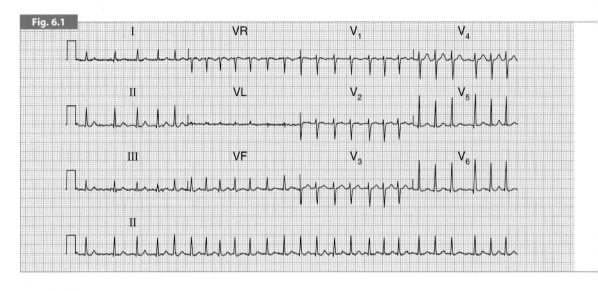

Fig. 6.1

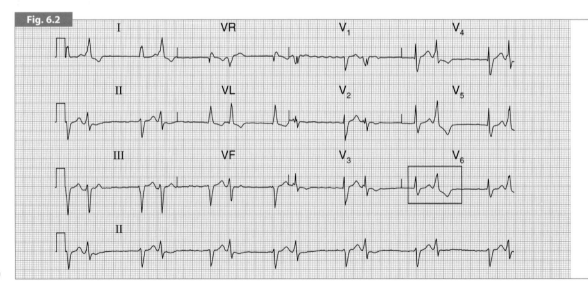

Fig. 6.2

Uncontrolled atrial fibrillation
Note
- Atrial fibrillation, with ventricular rate 170/min
- No other abnormalities
- No evidence of digoxin effect

RHYTHM PROBLEMS

A sudden rhythm change is a common cause of breathlessness, and even of frank pulmonary oedema. Arrhythmias can be paroxysmal, so the patient may be in sinus rhythm when examined, and a patient who is suddenly breathless may not be aware of an arrhythmia. When sudden breathlessness is associated with palpitations it is important to establish whether the breathlessness or the palpitations came first – palpitations following breathlessness may be due to the sinus tachycardia of anxiety. The ECG in Figure 6.1 is from a patient who developed pulmonary oedema due to the onset of uncontrolled atrial fibrillation.

Less dramatic rhythm abnormalities can also contribute to breathlessness, especially to breathlessness on exertion. This is true of both fast and slow rhythms. The ECG in Figure 6.2 is from a patient who had atrial fibrillation but who was breathless on exercise – partly because of coupled ventricular extrasystoles, which markedly reduced cardiac output as a result of an effective halving of the heart rate.

Atrial fibrillation with coupled ventricular extrasystoles
Note
- Atrial fibrillation, with slow and regular ventricular response
- Coupled ventricular extrasystoles
- In supraventricular beats, leads V$_5$–V$_6$ show a deep wide S wave, suggesting right bundle branch block
- ?Digoxin toxicity

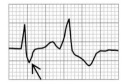

Deep wide S wave in supraventricular beat in lead V$_6$

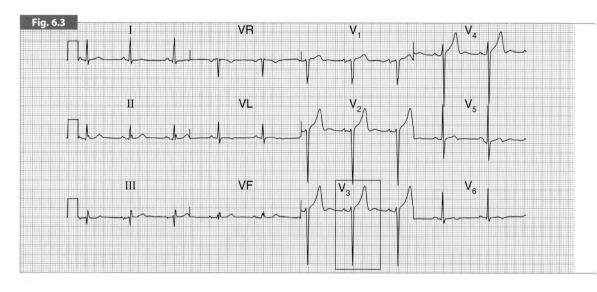

Fig. 6.3

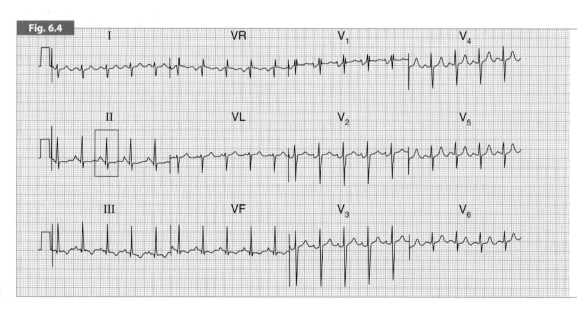

Fig. 6.4

Left atrial hypertrophy and left ventricular hypertrophy

Note

- Sinus rhythm
- Bifid P waves
- Normal axis
- Tall QRS complexes
- Inverted T waves in lead V_6, suggesting left ventricular hypertrophy

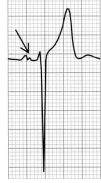

Bifid P wave in lead V_3

Mitral stenosis and pulmonary hypertension

Note

- Sinus rhythm
- Bifid P wave (best seen in lead II)
- Right axis deviation
- Partial right bundle branch block pattern
- Persistent S wave in lead V_6

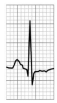

Bifid P wave in lead II

THE ECG IN DISORDERS AFFECTING THE LEFT SIDE OF THE HEART

THE ECG IN LEFT ATRIAL HYPERTROPHY

Left atrial hypertrophy causes a double (bifid) P wave. Left atrial hypertrophy without left ventricular hypertrophy is classically due to mitral stenosis, so the bifid P wave is sometimes called 'P mitrale'. This is misleading, because most patients whose ECGs have bifid P waves either have left ventricular hypertrophy that is not obvious on the ECG or – and perhaps this is more common – have a perfectly normal heart. The bifid P wave is thus not a useful measure of left atrial hypertrophy.

Figure 6.3 shows an ECG with a bifid P wave indicating left atrial hypertrophy. This was confirmed by echocardiography in the patient, who also had concentric left ventricular hypertrophy due to hypertension.

Significant mitral stenosis usually – but not always – leads to atrial fibrillation, in which no P waves, bifid or otherwise, can be seen. Occasional patients, such as the one whose ECG is shown in Figure 6.4, develop pulmonary hypertension and remain in sinus rhythm. There is then a combination of a bifid P wave with evidence of right ventricular hypertrophy. This combination does allow a confident diagnosis of severe mitral stenosis.

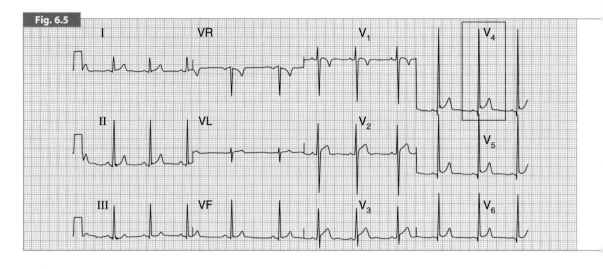

Fig. 6.5

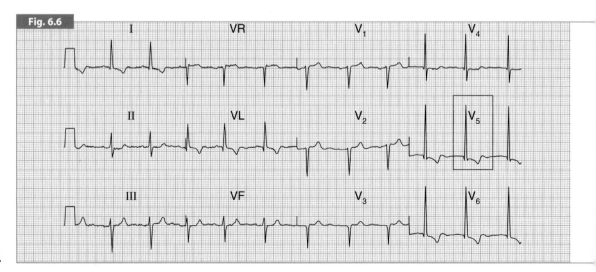

Fig. 6.6

Probably normal ECG

Note

- Sinus rhythm
- Normal axis
- Very tall R waves (meeting 'voltage criteria' for left ventricular hypertrophy)
- No other evidence of left ventricular hypertrophy

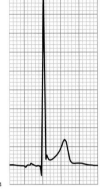

Tall R wave in lead V_4

Left ventricular hypertrophy

Note

- Sinus rhythm
- Voltage criteria for left ventricular hypertrophy
- Inverted T waves in leads I, VL, V_5–V_6

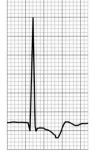

Tall R wave and inverted T wave in lead V_5

THE ECG IN LEFT VENTRICULAR HYPERTROPHY

Left ventricular hypertrophy may be caused by hypertension, aortic stenosis or incompetence, or mitral incompetence.

The ECG features of left ventricular hypertrophy are:

- an increased height of the QRS complex
- inverted T waves in the leads that 'look at' the left ventricle – I, VL and V_5–V_6.

Left axis deviation is not uncommon, but is due more to fibrosis causing left anterior hemiblock than to the left ventricular hypertrophy itself.

The ECG is a poor guide to the severity of left ventricular hypertrophy. Numerous criteria have been proposed that claim to detect the presence of left ventricular hypertrophy from ECG measurements. Most depend on measuring R or S waves in different leads, and some take the width of QRS complexes into account. The most commonly used indicators are the Sokolow–Lyon voltage criteria. These define left ventricular hypertrophy as being present when the depth of the S wave in lead V_1 plus the height of the R wave in lead V_5 or V_6 (whichever is the greater) exceeds 35 mm, although the S wave is usually also deep in lead V_2.

Unfortunately, voltage criteria have a low sensitivity as detectors of left ventricular hypertrophy, and are essentially useless. They would frequently lead to a diagnosis of left ventricular hypertrophy in perfectly healthy young men, even in those who are not athletic (Fig. 6.5).

The complete ECG picture of left ventricular hypertrophy is easy to recognize. The ECG in Figure 6.6 is from a patient with severe and untreated hypertension. It shows the 'voltage criteria' which, when combined with the T wave inversion in the lateral leads, probably are significant. In this case, the small Q waves in

295

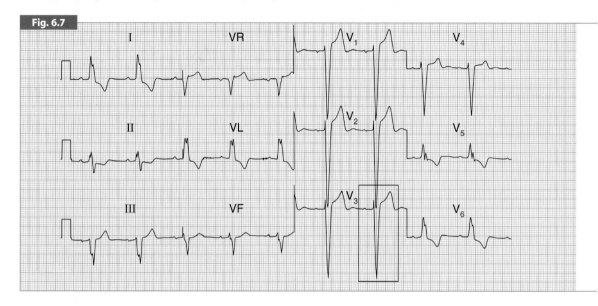

Fig. 6.7

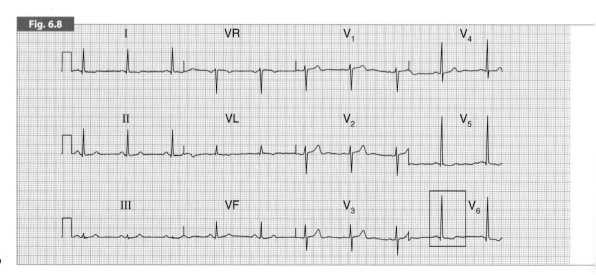

Fig. 6.8

Left bundle branch block with aortic stenosis

Note

- Sinus rhythm
- Normal axis
- Broad QRS complexes with LBBB pattern
- Very deep S waves in lead V_3
- Inverted T waves in leads I, VL, V_5–V_6

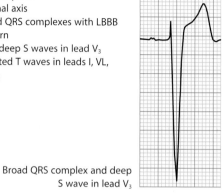

Broad QRS complex and deep S wave in lead V_3

Left ventricular hypertrophy

Note

- Sinus rhythm
- Normal axis
- Voltage criteria for left ventricular hypertrophy not met
- Inverted T waves in leads I, VL, V_6

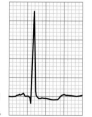

Normal R wave and inverted T wave in lead V_6

the lateral leads are septal and do not indicate a previous infarction. Note that the T wave inversion is most prominent in lead V_6, and becomes progressively less so in leads V_5 and V_4. This pattern of T wave inversion is sometimes referred to as 'left ventricular strain', but this is an old-fashioned and essentially meaningless term.

The most important cause of severe left ventricular hypertrophy is aortic valve disease: when aortic stenosis or incompetence causes left ventricular hypertrophy, aortic valve replacement must be considered. Aortic valve disease is frequently associated with left bundle branch block (LBBB) (Fig. 6.7), which completely masks any evidence of left ventricular hypertrophy. The patient who is breathless, or who has chest pain or dizziness, and has signs of aortic valve disease and an ECG showing LBBB, needs urgent investigation.

Unfortunately, the severity of ECG changes is an unreliable guide to the importance of the underlying cardiac problem. The ECG in Figure 6.8 shows lateral T wave inversion, but does not meet the 'voltage criteria', in a patient with moderate aortic stenosis (aortic valve gradient 60 mmHg).

In contrast, the ECG in Figure 6.9 is from a patient with severe aortic stenosis and an aortic valve gradient of > 120 mmHg, yet it shows little to suggest severe left ventricular hypertrophy.

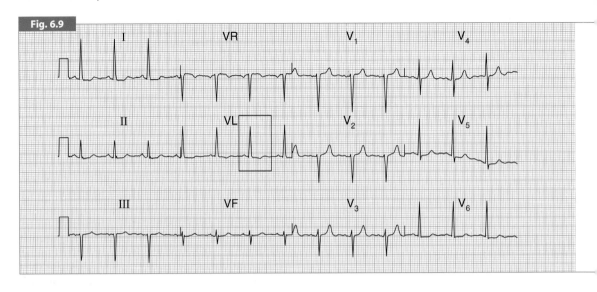

Fig. 6.9

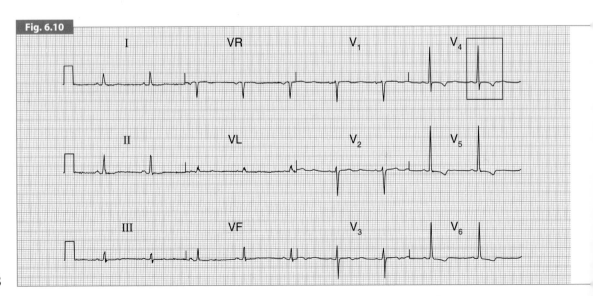

Fig. 6.10

?Left ventricular hypertrophy with severe aortic stenosis

Note
- Sinus rhythm
- Normal axis
- Voltage criteria for left ventricular hypertrophy not met
- Minor ST segment/T wave changes in leads I, VL, V₆

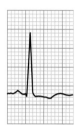

Minor ST segment/T wave changes in lead VL

Probable ischaemia

Note
- Sinus rhythm
- Normal axis
- T wave inversion in leads II and V₃–V₆, but most prominent in V₄–V₅

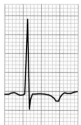

Inverted T wave in lead V₄

ECGs THAT CAN MIMIC LEFT VENTRICULAR HYPERTROPHY

The problems of differentiating between lateral T wave changes due to left ventricular hypertrophy and those due to ischaemia have been discussed in Chapter 5. The history and physical examination become extremely important, and the ECG must not be viewed in isolation. The ECG in Figure 6.10 is from a patient with chest pain that was compatible with, but not diagnostic of, angina and who had physical signs suggesting mild aortic stenosis. The T wave inversion is more prominent in leads V₄ and V₅ than in V₆, and is present in V₃. The T waves are upright in leads I and VL. These changes point to ischaemia rather than left ventricular hypertrophy, and ischaemia proved to be present in this patient.

The ECG in Figure 6.11 is from a patient with hypertension and breathlessness. He was shown to have left ventricular hypertrophy and coronary disease, but all the changes here could have been due to left ventricular hypertrophy alone.

When a breathless patient has an ECG with gross lateral T wave changes (Fig. 6.12), hypertrophic cardiomyopathy is a possibility (Box 6.4).

Lateral T wave changes associated with left anterior hemiblock often accompany left ventricular hypertrophy. However, there was no echocardiographic evidence of this in the patient whose ECG is shown in Figure 6.13. Here the changes must be due to conducting system disease.

Another example of a conducting tissue abnormality that could be mistaken for left ventricular hypertrophy is the Wolff–Parkinson–White (WPW) syndrome. The ECG in Figure 6.14 is from a young man with the WPW syndrome type B. There is left ventricular hypertrophy according to voltage criteria, and there is also lateral T wave inversion, but the diagnosis is made from the short PR intervals and the delta waves.

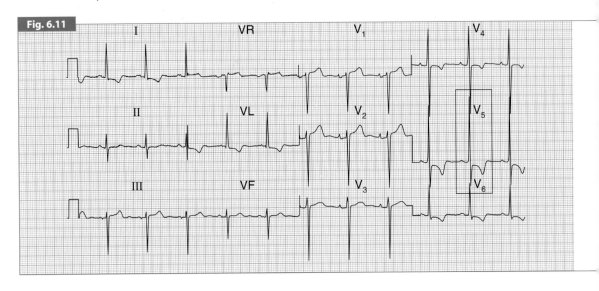

Fig. 6.11

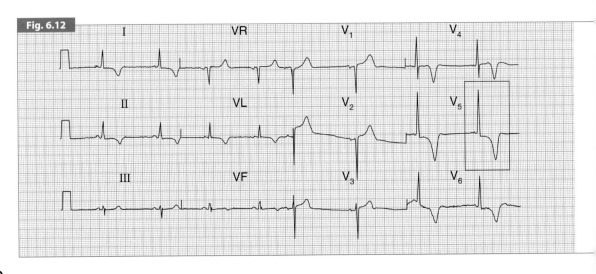

Fig. 6.12

?Left ventricular hypertrophy, ?ischaemia

Note
- Sinus rhythm
- Bifid P waves, best seen in lead I
- Normal axis
- T wave inversion in leads I, VL and V_3–V_6, but most prominent in V_5

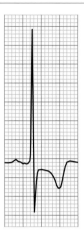

Maximal T wave inversion in lead V_5

Hypertrophic cardiomyopathy

Note
- Sinus rhythm
- Bifid P wave, best seen in lead V_4
- Voltage criteria for left ventricular hypertrophy not met
- Gross T wave inversion in leads V_4–V_6

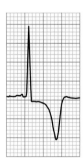

Normal R wave and dramatic T wave inversion in lead V_5

301

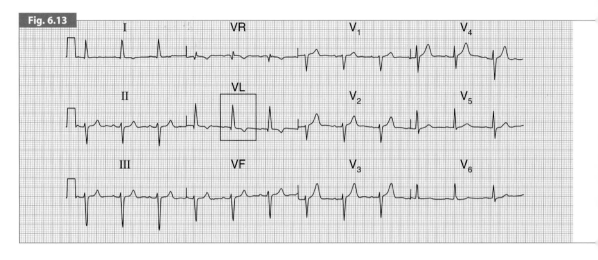

Fig. 6.13

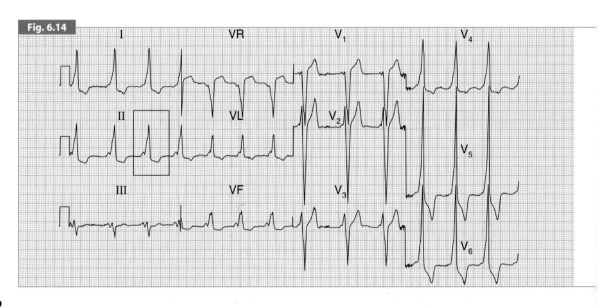

Fig. 6.14

Left anterior hemiblock

Note

- Sinus rhythm
- Left axis deviation
- Inverted T waves in leads I, VL

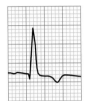

Inverted T wave in lead VL

The Wolff–Parkinson–White syndrome (no left ventricular hypertrophy)

Note

- Short PR interval
- Broad QRS complexes with delta waves
- Very tall R waves
- Inverted T waves in leads I, II, VL, V_4–V_6

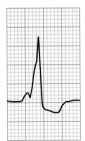

Short PR interval and delta wave in lead II

The height of the QRS complexes and the T wave inversion in this situation do not indicate left ventricular hypertrophy.

THE ECG IN DISORDERS AFFECTING THE RIGHT SIDE OF THE HEART

Right-sided heart disease can be the result of chronic lung disease (e.g. chronic obstructive airways disease, bronchiectasis), pulmonary embolism (especially when repeated episodes cause thromboembolic pulmonary hypertension), idiopathic pulmonary hypertension, or congenital heart disease. Any of these can cause right ventricular hypertrophy, but none of them causes a specific ECG abnormality (Boxes 6.7 and 6.8).

Box 6.7 **The ECG in pulmonary embolism**

- Sinus tachycardia
- Atrial arrhythmias
- Right atrial hypertrophy
- Right ventricular hypertrophy
- Right axis deviation
- Clockwise rotation, with persistent S wave in lead V_6
- Right bundle branch block
- Combination of S wave in lead I with Q wave and inverted T wave in lead III

Box 6.8 **The ECG in chronic obstructive pulmonary disease**

- Small QRS complexes
- Right atrial hypertrophy (P pulmonale)
- Right axis deviation
- Right ventricular hypertrophy
- Clockwise rotation, with persistent, deep S wave in lead V_6
- Right bundle branch block

303

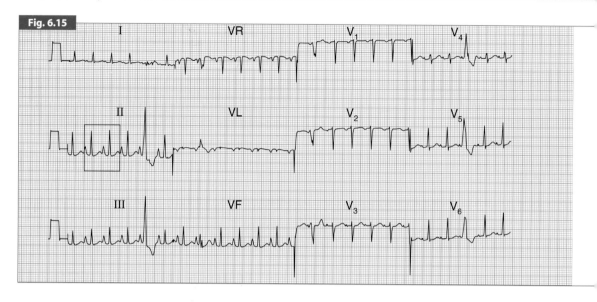

Fig. 6.15

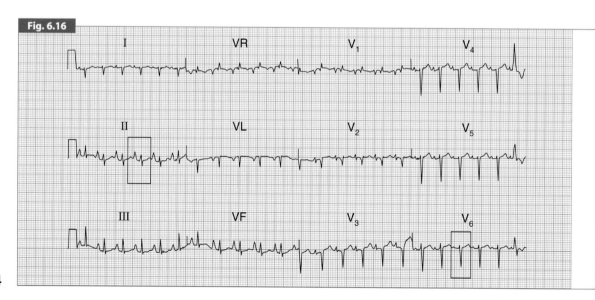

Fig. 6.16

Right atrial hypertrophy

Note

- Sinus rhythm with occasional aberrant conduction
- Tall and peaked P waves
- No other abnormality
- In this case the right atrial hypertrophy was due to tricuspid stenosis

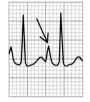

Peaked P wave in lead II

Right atrial and right ventricular hypertrophy

Note

- Peaked P waves, especially in lead II
- Right axis deviation
- Persistent S waves in lead V₆ (clockwise rotation) suggest chronic lung disease

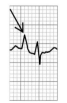 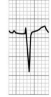

Peaked P wave
in lead II

Persistent S wave
in lead V₆

THE ECG IN RIGHT ATRIAL HYPERTROPHY

Right atrial hypertrophy causes tall and peaked P waves, which are sometimes described as 'P pulmonale'. There is, in fact, such variation within the normal range of P waves that the diagnosis of right atrial hypertrophy is difficult to make. Its presence can be inferred when peaked P waves are associated with the ECG changes of right ventricular hypertrophy. Evidence of right atrial hypertrophy without right ventricular hypertrophy will usually only be seen in patients with tricuspid stenosis (Fig. 6.15).

The ECG in Figure 6.16 is from a patient with right atrial and right ventricular hypertrophy due to severe chronic obstructive pulmonary disease.

THE ECG IN RIGHT VENTRICULAR HYPERTROPHY

The ECG changes associated with right ventricular hypertrophy are:

- right axis deviation
- a dominant R wave in lead V_1
- clockwise rotation of the heart: as the septum is displaced laterally, the transition of the QRS complex in the chest leads from a right to a left ventricular configuration occurs in leads V_4–V_6 instead of V_2–V_4; there is thus a persistent S wave in lead V_6, which normally does not show an S wave at all
- inversion of the T wave in leads that 'look at' the right ventricle: V_1, V_2 and occasionally V_3.

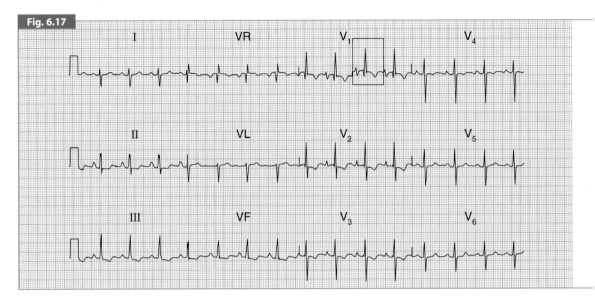

Fig. 6.17

Table 6.1 **Possible alternative causes of the ECG appearance of right ventricular hypertrophy**

ECG feature	Cause
Right axis deviation	Normal in tall thin people
Dominant R wave in lead V_1	Normal variant Posterior infarction The Wolff–Parkinson–White syndrome Right bundle branch block of any cause
Inverted T waves in leads V_1–V_2	Normal variant, especially in black people Anterior non-ST segment elevation myocardial infarction The Wolff–Parkinson–White syndrome Right bundle branch block of any cause Cardiomyopathy
Apparent clockwise rotation	Dextrocardia

Marked right ventricular hypertrophy

Note

- Sinus rhythm
- Peaked P waves
- Right axis deviation
- Dominant R waves in lead V$_1$
- Persistent S waves in lead V$_6$

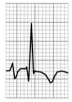

Dominant R wave in lead V$_1$

In extreme cases it is easy to diagnose right ventricular hypertrophy from the ECG. The ECG in Figure 6.17 came from a patient incapacitated by breathlessness due to primary pulmonary hypertension.

As with the ECG in left ventricular hypertrophy, none of the ECG changes of right ventricular hypertrophy individually provide unequivocal evidence of right ventricular hypertrophy (Table 6.1). Conversely, it is possible to have marked right ventricular hypertrophy without all the typical ECG features being present. Minor degrees of right axis deviation are seen in normal people, and a dominant R wave in lead V$_1$ is occasionally seen in normal people, although it is never more than 3 or 4 mm tall. A dominant R wave in lead V$_1$ may also indicate a 'true posterior' myocardial infarction (see Ch. 5). There may be

variation in the T wave inversion in leads V$_1$ and V$_2$ in normal subjects (see Ch. 1) and, particularly in black people, the T wave can be inverted in leads V$_2$ and V$_3$.

The ECG in Figure 6.18 shows a dominant R wave in lead V$_1$ but no other evidence of right ventricular hypertrophy. This could indicate a posterior myocardial infarction (see Ch. 5), but this trace was from a young man who was asymptomatic, who had no abnormalities on examination, and whose echocardiogram was normal. This is a normal variant.

The ECG in Figure 6.19 is from a young woman who had become progressively more breathless since the birth of her baby 4 months previously. She had had no chest pain. No previous ECGs were available. The anterior T wave changes could be a normal variant in a black woman. T wave inversion in leads V$_3$–V$_4$ could indicate anterior ischaemia, but the important point here is that the T wave inversion is most prominent in leads V$_1$–V$_2$, and becomes progressively less in V$_3$–V$_4$. This is characteristic of T wave inversion due to right ventricular hypertrophy. In this case the T wave inversion, combined with right axis deviation and a persistent S wave in lead V$_6$, suggests right ventricular hypertrophy. The patient was shown to have had recurrent small pulmonary emboli.

A prominent S wave in lead V$_6$ is sometimes called 'persistent' because this lead should show a pure left ventricular type of complex with a dominant R wave and no S wave. The 'transition point', when the R and S waves are equal, indicates the position of the interventricular septum and this is normally under the position of lead V$_3$ or V$_4$. In the ECG in Figure 6.20 a transition point is not present at all, and lead V$_6$ shows a small R wave and a dominant S wave. This is due to the right ventricle underlying more of the precordium than usual. This change is characteristic of chronic lung disease.

307

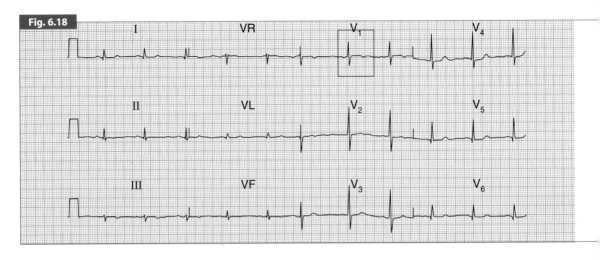

Fig. 6.18

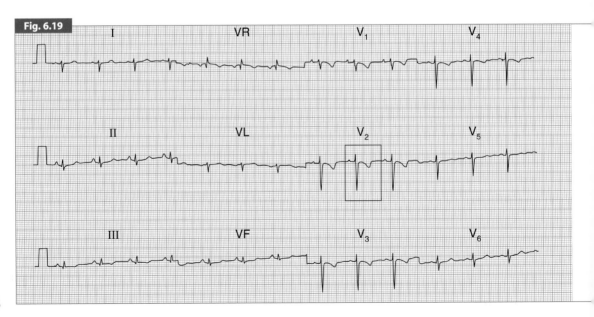

Fig. 6.19

Probable normal variant

Note
- Sinus rhythm
- Normal axis
- Dominant R waves in lead V_1
- Inverted T waves in lead III

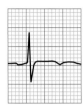

Dominant R wave in lead V_1

Right ventricular hypertrophy

Note
- Sinus rhythm
- Right axis deviation
- No dominant R waves in lead V_1
- Inverted T waves in leads V_1–V_4, maximal in lead V_1
- Persistent S waves in lead V_6

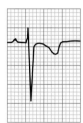

Inverted T wave in lead V_2

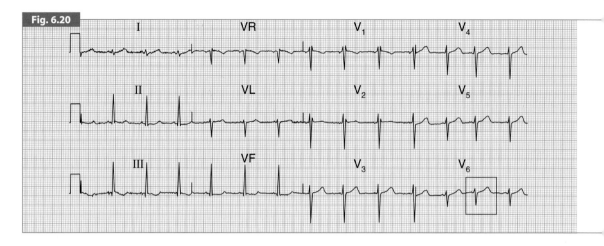

Fig. 6.20

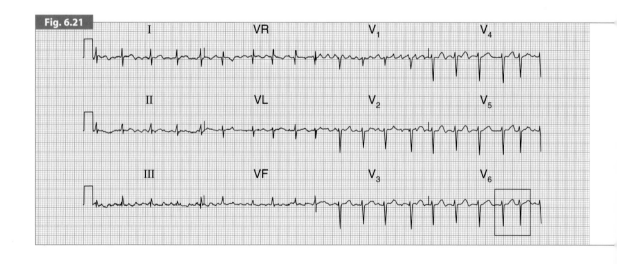

Fig. 6.21

Chronic lung disease

Note

- Sinus rhythm
- Right axis deviation
- Prominent S waves in lead V_6
- Nonspecific T wave changes in leads III and VF

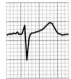

Persistent S wave in lead V_6

When breathlessness is accompanied by a sudden change in rotation, a pulmonary embolus is likely. The ECG in Figure 6.21 is from a patient who had had a normal preoperative ECG but who developed breathlessness with atrial fibrillation a week after cholecystectomy. The deep S wave in lead V_6 is the pointer towards a pulmonary embolus being the cause of the atrial fibrillation.

As with the ECG in left ventricular hypertrophy, it is the appearance of changes in serial recordings that provides the best evidence of minor or moderate degrees of right ventricular hypertrophy. In the majority of cases in which the ECG suggests right ventricular hypertrophy, it is not possible to diagnose the underlying disease process with certainty.

?Pulmonary embolus

Note

- Atrial fibrillation, ventricular rate 114/min
- Dominant S wave in lead V_6
- No other evidence of right ventricular hypertrophy

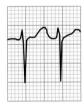

Persistent S wave in lead V_6

WHAT TO DO ▶

In most patients with breathlessness, the ECG does not contribute very much to diagnosis and management, and the important thing is to treat the patient and not the ECG.

The ECG cannot diagnose heart failure, although heart failure is unlikely if the ECG is totally normal. By demonstrating ischaemia or enlargement of one or more of the cardiac chambers, the ECG may help to identify the underlying disease that requires treatment. However, the symptoms of acute heart failure need empirical treatment whatever the ECG shows, and this should not be delayed while an ECG is being recorded.

The ECG can provide confirmatory evidence that breathlessness is due to a pulmonary embolus or chronic lung disease, but it is an unreliable way of making this diagnosis and treatment cannot depend on the ECG. Similarly, the ECG will not help in the diagnosis of anaemia, though it may show ischaemic changes.

In general then, the management of the breathless patient does not depend on the ECG unless breathlessness is due to heart failure which is secondary to an arrhythmia. In that case, the ECG is essential both for diagnosis and for monitoring the response to therapy.

CARDIAC RESYNCHRONIZATION THERAPY (CRT)

Patients with severe heart failure, especially those whose ECG shows left bundle branch block with a broad QRS complex, may have dyssynchronous cardiac contraction. Instead of both sides of the left ventricle contracting simultaneously in systole, there is a substantial delay between contraction of the left ventricular septum and the free wall. This reduces the stroke volume and exacerbates the heart failure. Contraction can be resynchronized by pacing the left ventricular free wall and the septum simultaneously. This is achieved by two pacing leads – one placed in a branch of the coronary sinus (the venous side of the coronary circulation, which drains into the right atrium), with a second, right ventricular, lead to pace the septum. This technique, 'cardiac resynchronization therapy' (CRT), is also known as biventricular pacing, or simply 'bivent'. Resynchronization improves both cardiac output and symptomatic heart failure. In addition to right ventricular and coronary sinus leads, there will usually be an atrial lead if sinus rhythm is present, because atrial systole may make an important contribution to cardiac output (Fig. 6.22).

INDICATIONS FOR CRT

Numerous clinical studies have shown that, in appropriate patients, CRT can improve left ventricular function and ejection fraction, and can improve exercise capacity. In patients still symptomatic from heart failure despite optimal medical therapy, CRT has been shown to reduce morbidity and all-cause mortality. CRT is therefore now considered a standard therapy; its indications are listed in Box 6.9. However, its role

Box 6.9 Indications for cardiac resynchronization therapy

These remain uncertain, but it is currently recommended for patients:
- on optimal pharmacotherapy and
- with an ejection fraction of less than 35% and
- with left bundle branch block with a QRS complex longer than 150 ms (or 120–149 ms and with echocardiographic evidence of dyssynchrony) and
- with heart failure symptoms in NYHA Class III or IV

Fig. 6.22

Chest X-ray showing biventricular pacemaker

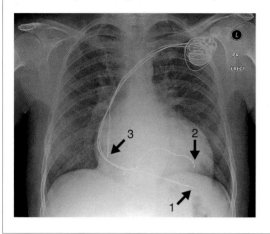

Note
- Ventricular lead in right ventricular apex position (arrow 1)
- Coronary sinus lead for left ventricular pacing (arrow 2)
- Atrial lead in right atrial appendage position (arrow 3)

in patients with less severe symptoms, or with atrial fibrillation or pacemaker dependence, has not been established. Since it is an invasive and costly procedure, patient selection is clearly extremely important.

ECG APPEARANCE

Biventricular pacing needs to be continuous, or 'obligate' (as opposed to 'on demand'), because resynchronization cannot be achieved unless the heart is in a paced rhythm. If necessary, pacing is ensured by careful programming of the AV delay or by pharmacological suppression of the intrinsic rhythm.

The pacing spike may be complex and may have two components. The QRS complex of the paced beat may have either a narrowed left bundle branch block morphology or a right bundle branch block morphology (Fig. 6.23).

Patients without an atrial lead will usually have atrial fibrillation or atrial flutter.

SPECIALIST FUNCTIONS

Patients with severe left ventricular dysfunction are at increased risk of ventricular arrhythmias, so some CRT devices incorporate a ventricular implanted cardioverter defibrillation element (CRTD). This device will function in the same way as a conventional biventricular pacing device, but with the additional function of an ICD (see Ch. 3).

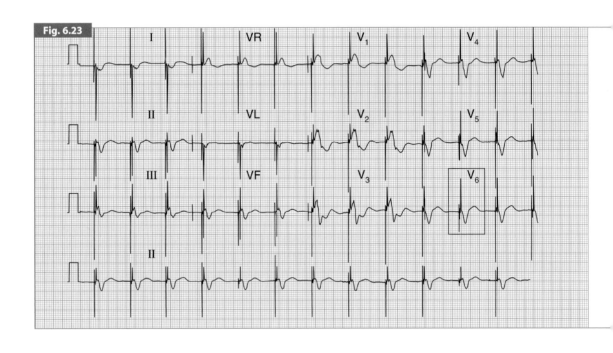

Fig. 6.23

Biventricular pacing

Note

- Complex ventricular pacing spike, sometimes with two distinct elements derived from the right ventricular and coronary sinus leads
- Right bundle branch block morphology in the QRS complexes
- Obligate pacing throughout

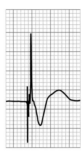

Two juxtaposed pacing spikes

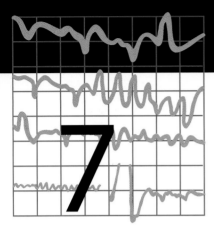

7

The effects of other conditions on the ECG

Artefacts in ECG recordings   316

The ECG in congenital heart disease   320

The ECG in systemic diseases   327

The effects of serum electrolyte
abnormalities on the ECG   331

The effects of medication on the ECG   335

Other causes of an abnormal ECG   343

The ECG is not a good method for investigating or diagnosing any condition that is not primarily cardiac. However, some generalized diseases do affect the ECG:

it is important to recognize this, and not assume that a patient has heart disease simply because their ECG seems abnormal.

ARTEFACTS IN ECG RECORDINGS

THE EFFECTS OF ABNORMAL MUSCLE MOVEMENT

Although ECG recorders are designed to be especially sensitive to the electrical frequencies of cardiac muscle contraction, the ECG will also record the contraction of skeletal muscles. The most common pattern of 'ECG abnormality' is a high-frequency oscillation due to general muscular tension in a patient who is not properly relaxed.

Fig. 7.1

Parkinsonism

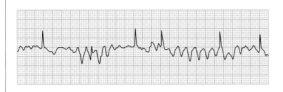

Note
- Muscle tremor at 5/s gives an appearance resembling atrial flutter
- The irregular QRS complexes may indicate that the rhythm is actually atrial fibrillation
- This record demonstrates the importance of looking at the patient as well as the ECG

Sustained involuntary tremors, such as those associated with Parkinsonism (Fig. 7.1) cause rhythmic ECG abnormalities that may be confused with cardiac arrhythmias.

HYPOTHERMIA

Hypothermia causes shivering, and therefore artefacts due to muscular activity. However, there can be other changes in the ECG, and the characteristic ECG feature of hypothermia is the 'J' wave. This is a small hump seen at the end of the QRS complex (Fig. 7.2).

The ECG in Figure 7.2 was recorded from a 76-year-old woman who was admitted to hospital with a temperature of 30°C after lying for a prolonged period in a freezing house, after a fall. She initially had a heart rate of 26/min, and the rhythm was atrial flutter. J waves can be seen in the lateral chest leads. On re-warming, she began to shiver, and, despite the muscle artefact, her heart can be seen to have reverted to sinus rhythm with first degree block. J waves are still visible (Fig. 7.3). When her temperature had returned to normal, the PR interval normalized and the J waves disappeared (Fig. 7.4).

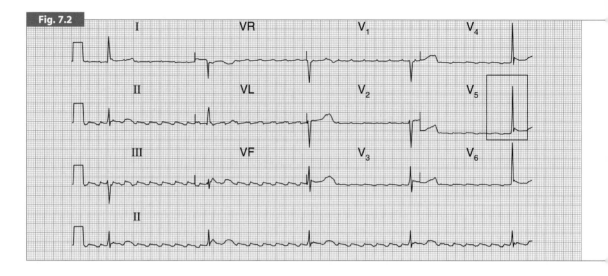

Fig. 7.2

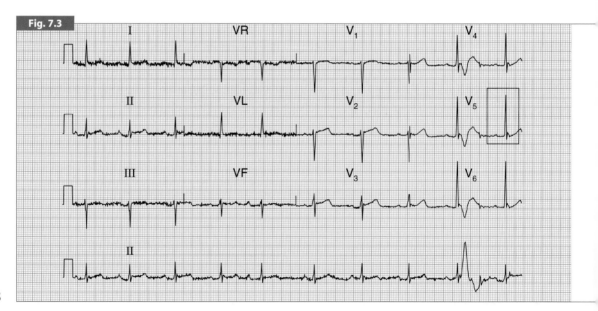

Fig. 7.3

Atrial flutter, hypothermia
Note
- Atrial flutter with ventricular rate 26/min
- J waves visible in leads V_4–V_6

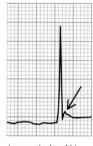

J wave in lead V_5

Hypothermia
Note
- Same patient as in Figures 7.2 and 7.4
- Sinus rhythm is restored
- The patient has begun to shiver (muscle artefact in the limb leads, with a further artefact in the penultimate complex of the rhythm strip)
- First degree block
- J waves still visible

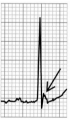

J wave in lead V_5

Fig. 7.4

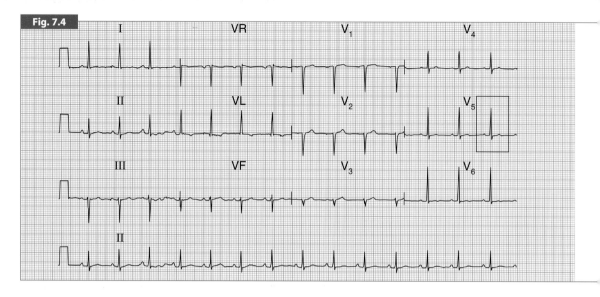

THE ECG IN CONGENITAL HEART DISEASE

The ECG provides a limited amount of help in the diagnosis of congenital heart disease by showing which chambers of the heart are enlarged. It is important to remember (see Ch. 1) that at birth the ECG of a normal infant shows a pattern of 'right ventricular hypertrophy', and this gradually disappears during the first 2 years of life.

If the infant pattern persists beyond the age of 2 years, right ventricular hypertrophy is indeed present. If there is a left ventricular, or normal adult, pattern before this age, then left ventricular hypertrophy is probably present. In older children the criteria for left and right ventricular hypertrophy are the same as in adults.

Box 7.1 lists some common congenital disorders and the associated ECG appearances.

Re-warming after hypothermia

Note

- Same patient as in Figures 7.2 and 7.3
- The patient is now in sinus rhythm with a normal PR interval
- J waves have disappeared
- There are some nonspecific ST segment and T wave

changes in leads I–II, VL, V$_6$

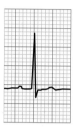

No J wave in lead V$_5$

Box 7.1 **ECG appearance in common congenital disorders**

Right ventricular hypertrophy
- Pulmonary hypertension of any cause (e.g. Eisenmenger's syndrome)
- Severe pulmonary stenosis
- Fallot's tetralogy
- Transposition of the great arteries

Left ventricular hypertrophy
- Aortic stenosis
- Coarctation of the aorta
- Mitral regurgitation
- Obstructive cardiomyopathy

Biventricular hypertrophy
- Ventricular septal defect

Right atrial hypertrophy
- Tricuspid stenosis

Right bundle branch block
- Atrial septal defect
- Complex defects

Left axis deviation
- Endocardial cushion defects
- Corrected transposition

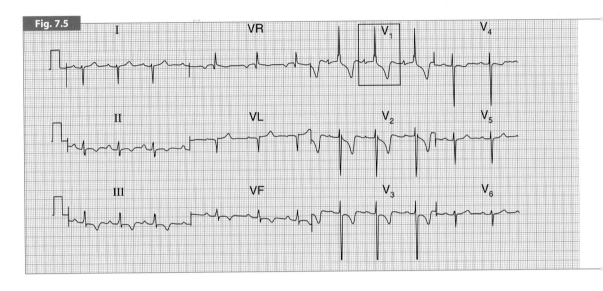

Fig. 7.5

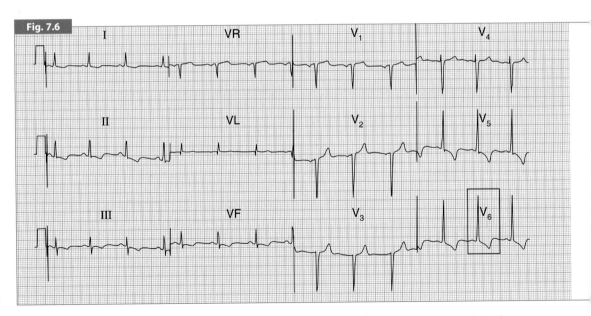

Fig. 7.6

Pulmonary stenosis

Note

- Sinus rhythm
- Right axis deviation
- Dominant R waves in lead V_1
- Persistent S waves in lead V_6
- Inverted T waves in leads V_1–V_4

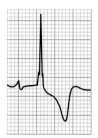

Dominant R wave in lead V_1

The ECG in Figure 7.5 shows all the features of severe right ventricular hypertrophy: it came from a boy with severe pulmonary stenosis.

The ECG in Figure 7.6 shows left ventricular hypertrophy, and was recorded in an 8-year-old with severe aortic stenosis.

Left ventricular hypertrophy

Note

- Sinus rhythm
- Normal axis
- Left ventricular hypertrophy according to voltage criteria
- T wave inversion in leads I, V_5–V_6

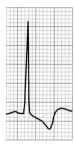

Tall R wave and inverted T wave in lead V_6

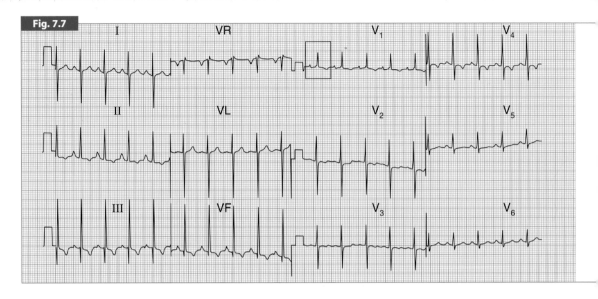

Fig. 7.7

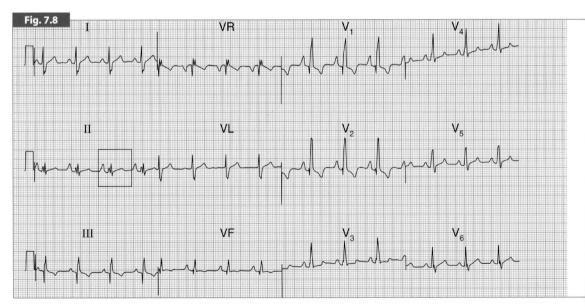

Fig. 7.8

Right ventricular hypertrophy in Fallot's tetralogy

Note

- Leads V_1–V_6 recorded at half sensitivity
- Sinus rhythm
- Right axis deviation
- Dominant R waves in lead V_1
- T wave inversion in leads II–III, VF, V_1–V_4

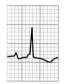

Dominant R wave in lead V_1

The ECG in Figure 7.7 shows right ventricular hypertrophy, and came from a young woman who had had a partial correction of Fallot's tetralogy 20 years previously.

The ECG in Figure 7.8 suggests right atrial hypertrophy and shows right bundle branch block. It came from a teenager with Ebstein's anomaly and an atrial septal defect.

Right atrial hypertrophy and right bundle branch block, in Ebstein's anomaly

Note

- Sinus rhythm
- Peaked P waves in lead II
- Broad QRS complexes with right bundle branch block pattern

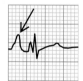

Peaked P wave in lead II

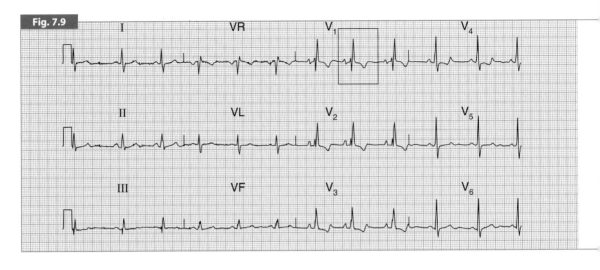

Fig. 7.9

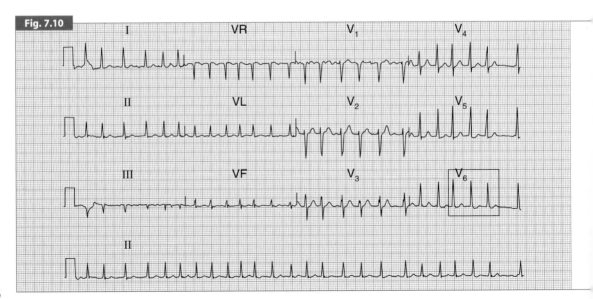

Fig. 7.10

Right bundle branch block with atrial septal defect
Note
- Sinus rhythm
- Normal axis
- QRS complex duration within normal limits (108 ms)
- RBBB pattern

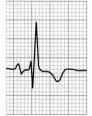

RBBB pattern in lead V$_1$

It is usually fairly obvious that a patient has congenital heart disease of some sort, but the condition that may be missed is an atrial septal defect. The ECG in Figure 7.9 is from a 50-year-old woman who complained of mild but increasing breathlessness. She had a rather nonspecific systolic murmur at the left sternal edge. Her GP recorded an ECG which showed right bundle branch block, and as a result she had an echocardiogram which showed an atrial septal defect.

THE ECG IN SYSTEMIC DISEASES

Cardiac involvement in a generalized disorder can cause arrhythmias and conduction defects, particularly if there is infiltration or the deposition of abnormal substances in the myocardium.

THYROID DISEASE

Thyrotoxicosis is probably the most common noncardiac disorder that may present as a cardiac problem. It may cause atrial fibrillation, particularly in old age. There is usually a rapid ventricular response, which is difficult to control with digoxin (Fig. 7.10). An elderly patient may complain of palpitations or the symptoms of heart failure, and arterial embolization may occur. The usual symptoms of thyrotoxicosis may be mild or even absent.

Thyrotoxicosis
Note
- Atrial fibrillation
- Ventricular rate 153/min
- Some ST segment depression in leads V$_5$–V$_6$: ?digoxin effect
- No other abnormalities

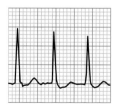

Rapid ventricular rate in lead V$_6$

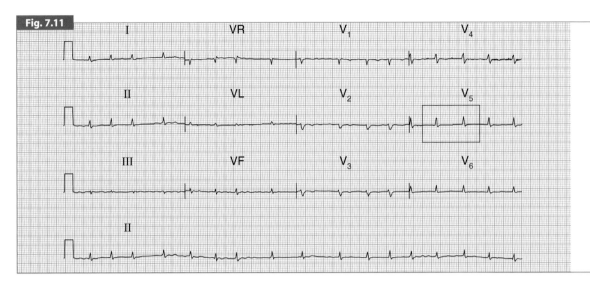

Fig. 7.11

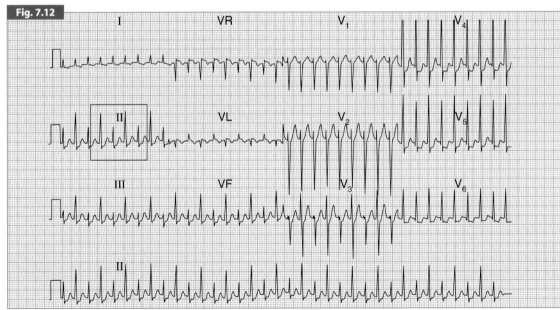

Fig. 7.12

Malignant pericardial effusion

Note

- Atrial fibrillation
- Generally small QRS complexes
- Widespread T wave flattening

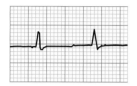

Small QRS complexes and flat T waves in lead V₅

MALIGNANCY

Metastatic deposits in and around the heart can cause virtually any arrhythmia or conduction disturbance. Malignancy is the most common cause of a large pericardial effusion, and a combination of atrial fibrillation and small complexes on the ECG suggest a malignant pericardial effusion. The ECG in Figure 7.11 is from a 60-year-old man with metastatic bronchial carcinoma.

In the case of large pericardial effusions, with each beat the heart can rock within the effusion, causing alternate large and small QRS complexes. This is called 'electrical alternans'. The ECG in Figure 7.12 is from another patient with carcinoma of the bronchus, who presented with a supraventricular tachycardia. Electrical alternans suggests the presence of a pericardial effusion, though in this case the QRS complexes are of normal size.

Electrical alternans

Note

- Narrow complex tachycardia at 200/min (AVRNT)
- Alternate large and small QRS complexes

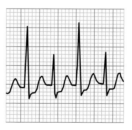

Alternate large and small QRS complexes in lead II

Box 7.2 Causes of electrolyte imbalance

Hyperkalaemia
- Renal failure
- Potassium-retaining diuretics (amiloride, spironolactone, triamterene)
- Angiotensin-converting enzyme inhibitors
- Liquorice
- Bartter's syndrome

Hypokalaemia
- Diuretic therapy
- Antidiuretic hormone secretion

Hypercalcaemia
- Hyperparathyroidism
- Renal failure

- Sarcoidosis
- Malignancy
- Myeloma
- Excess vitamin D
- Thiazide diuretics

Hypocalcaemia
- Hypoparathyroidism
- Severe diarrhoea
- Enteric fistulae
- Alkalosis
- Vitamin D deficiency

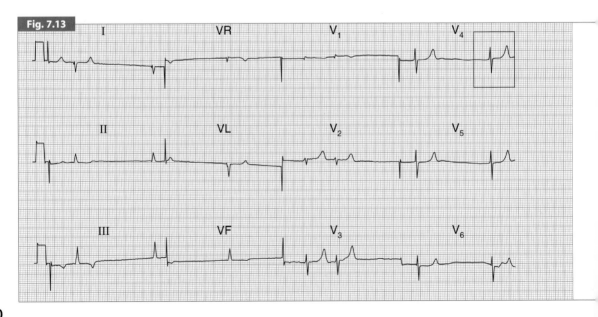

Fig. 7.13

Table 7.1 The effects of electrolyte imbalance on the ECG

Electrolyte	Effect of abnormal serum electrolyte level on ECG	
	Low level	High level
Potassium or magnesium	Flat T waves Prominent U waves Depressed ST segment Prolonged QT interval First or second degree block	Flat P waves Widening of QRS complexes (nonspecific intraventricular conduction delay) Tall peaked T waves Disappearance of ST segment Arrhythmias
Calcium	Prolonged QT interval (due to long ST segment)	Short QT interval, with loss of ST segment

Hyperkalaemia
Note
- No P waves
- ?Atrial fibrillation
- ?Junctional escape rhythm
- Right axis deviation
- Symmetrically peaked T waves, especially in the chest leads
- Inverted T waves in leads III, VF

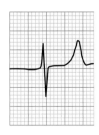

P wave absent and peaked T wave in lead V$_4$

THE EFFECTS OF SERUM ELECTROLYTE ABNORMALITIES ON THE ECG

Although abnormal levels of serum potassium, magnesium and calcium can affect the ECG, the 'classical' changes are rarely seen. Occasionally an ECG may suggest that the electrolytes should be checked, but the range of normality in the ECG is so great that an ECG is an unrealistic guide to electrolyte balance. Box 7.2 lists possible causes of electrolyte imbalance, and Table 7.1 summarizes the ECG changes that may occur.

POTASSIUM

Hyperkalaemia may cause arrhythmias, including ventricular fibrillation or asystole; flattening of the P waves; widening of the QRS complexes; depression or loss of the ST segment; and, particularly, symmetrical peaking of the T waves. The ECG in Figure 7.13 is from a

331

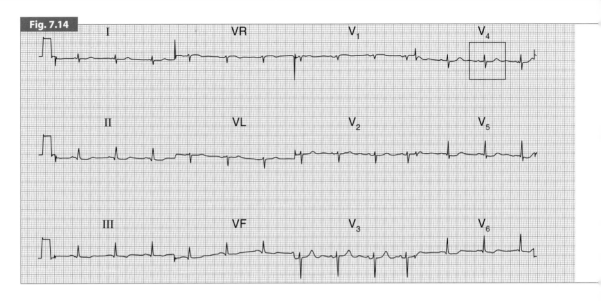

Fig. 7.14

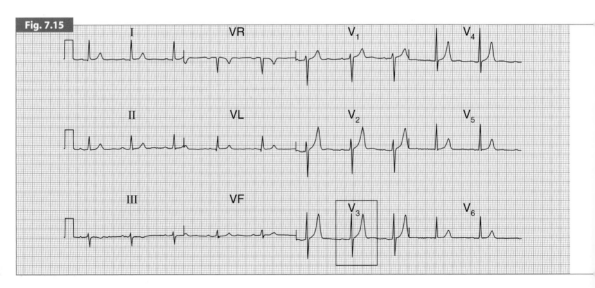

Fig. 7.15

Hyperkalaemia corrected

Note

- Same patient as in Figure 7.13
- Sinus rhythm
- ST segment depression in inferior lateral leads
- Normal T wave configuration

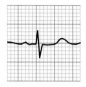

Normal P and T waves in lead V₄

patient with renal failure and a potassium level of 7.4 mmol. After correction of the plasma potassium level, sinus rhythm was restored and the T waves were no longer peaked (Fig. 7.14).

Remember, however, that peaked T waves are also a common finding in completely healthy patients (Fig. 7.15).

Normal ECG

Note

- Sinus rhythm
- Normal axis
- Tall peaked T waves, resembling hyperkalaemia

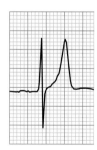

Tall, peaked T wave in lead V₃

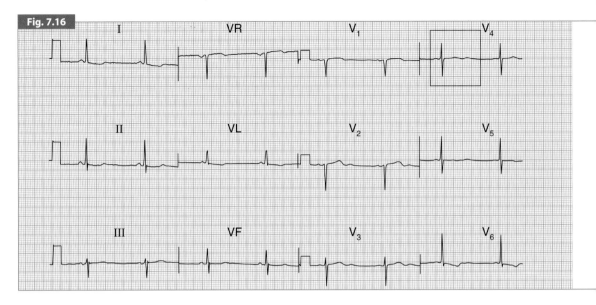

Fig. 7.16

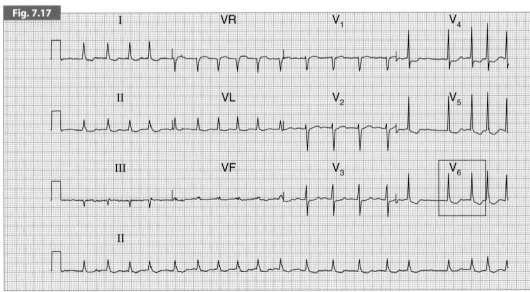

Fig. 7.17

Hypokalaemia
Note
- Leads V_1–V_6 recorded at half sensitivity
- Atrial fibrillation
- Normal axis
- Normal QRS complexes
- Flat T waves, with U waves in leads V_4–V_5

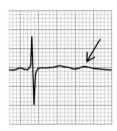

U wave in lead V_4

Digoxin effect
Note
- Atrial fibrillation
- Normal axis
- Normal QRS complexes
- Downward-sloping ST segments in leads V_5–V_6

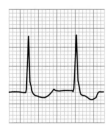

Downward-sloping ST segment in lead V_6

Hypokalaemia is common in patients with cardiac disease who are treated with powerful diuretics. It causes flattening of the T waves, prolongation of the QT interval, and the appearance of U waves. The ECG in Figure 7.16 was recorded from a patient with severe heart failure due to ischaemic heart disease. The serum potassium level fell to 1.9 mmol, as a result of loop diuretic treatment without either potassium supplementation or the concomitant administration of an angiotensin-converting enzyme inhibitor.

MAGNESIUM

The effects of high and low serum magnesium levels on the ECG are essentially the same as those of high and low potassium levels.

CALCIUM

Hypercalcaemia shortens, and hypocalcaemia prolongs, the QT interval. However, the ECG remains normal within a very wide range of serum calcium levels.

THE EFFECTS OF MEDICATION ON THE ECG

DIGOXIN

Atrial fibrillation is normally associated with a rapid ventricular response (sometimes inappropriately called 'fast AF'), unless conduction through the atrioventricular node is slowed by medication. Digoxin is still the best drug for controlling the ventricular rate in atrial fibrillation. The dose can be critical: the first sign of toxicity is a loss of appetite, and then the patient feels sick and vomits. Rarely, the patient complains of seeing yellow (xanthopsia). The main effect of digoxin on the ECG is downward sloping of the ST segments, especially in the lateral leads. The appearance is sometimes referred to as a 'reverse tick' (Fig. 7.17).

335

Fig. 7.18

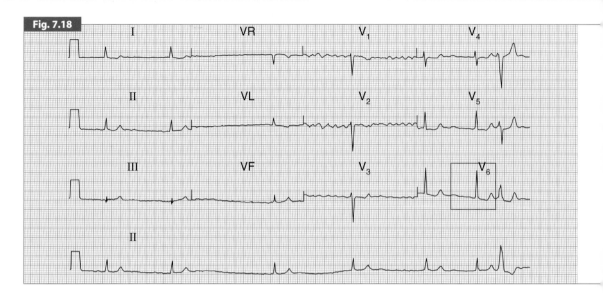

Fig. 7.19

Digoxin toxicity

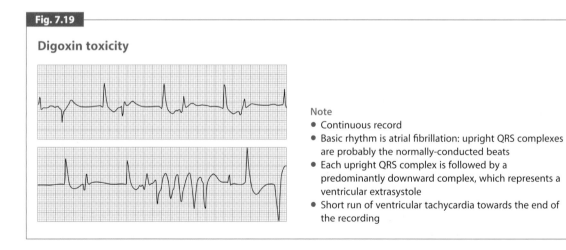

Note
- Continuous record
- Basic rhythm is atrial fibrillation: upright QRS complexes are probably the normally-conducted beats
- Each upright QRS complex is followed by a predominantly downward complex, which represents a ventricular extrasystole
- Short run of ventricular tachycardia towards the end of the recording

Digoxin toxicity

Note
- Atrial fibrillation with one ventricular extrasystole
- Ventricular rate 41/min
- Normal QRS complexes
- Digoxin effect on ST segments in lead V_6

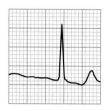

Downward-sloping ST segment in lead V_6

With increasing doses of digoxin the ventricular rate becomes regular and slow, and eventually complete heart block may develop. Digoxin can cause almost any arrhythmia, but especially ventricular extrasystoles and sometimes ventricular tachycardia. There is only a loose correlation between the symptoms and the ECG signs of digoxin toxicity.

The ECG in Figure 7.18 was recorded from a patient with a congestive cardiomyopathy which caused atrial fibrillation and heart failure. She was vomiting and her failure had deteriorated, her heart rate having fallen to about 40 beats/min.

The ECG in Figure 7.19 shows another example of digoxin toxicity, which caused syncopal attacks due to runs of ventricular tachycardia.

The effects of digoxin on the ECG are listed in Box 7.3.

Box 7.3 Effects of digoxin on the ECG

- Downward sloping ST segments
- Flattened or inverted T waves
- Short QT interval
- Almost any abnormal cardiac rhythm, but especially:
  — sinus bradycardia
  — paroxysmal atrial tachycardia with AV block
  — ventricular extrasystoles
  — ventricular tachycardia
  — any degree of AV block
- Regularization of QRS complexes in atrial fibrillation suggests toxicity

DRUGS THAT PROLONG THE QT INTERVAL

Over 200 drugs have been claimed to cause QT interval prolongation or torsade de pointes ventricular tachycardia (TdP VT). This is particularly true of the Class I and Class III antiarrhythmic drugs. It is sensible to regard all antiarrhythmic drugs as being potentially pro-arrhythmic, with the exception of the beta-blockers other than sotalol. While TdP VT is most commonly seen in patients whose ECGs have a prolonged QT interval, in some individuals the two are apparently not related. The ECG in Figure 7.20 was recorded from a patient treated with amiodarone; the T wave changes disappeared when the drug was discontinued.

Some of the more commonly used drugs which may cause QT interval prolongation and have been associated with TdP VT are listed in Box 7.4.

Several drugs that were otherwise very useful have been withdrawn because of the problems of QT interval prolongation and TdP VT. The list includes the gastric pro-motility agent cisapride, the antihistamine terfenadine, the antiplatelet agent ketanserin and the vasodilator prenylamine.

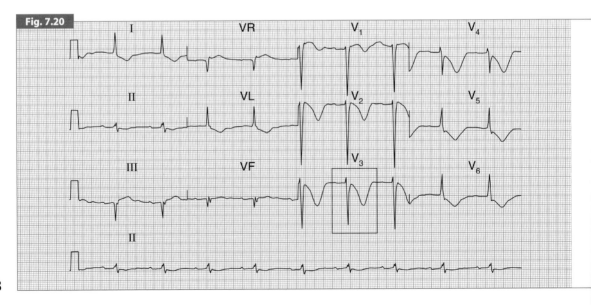

Fig. 7.20

Box 7.4 Drugs associated with QT interval prolongation and torsade de pointes ventricular tachycardia

Antiarrhythmic drugs
- Amiodarone
- Disopyramide
- Flecainide
- Procainamide
- Propafenone
- Quinidine (of historical interest only)
- Sotalol

Psychiatric drugs
- Amitriptyline
- Chlorpromazine
- Citalopram
- Doxepin
- Haloperidol
- Imipramine
- Lithium
- Prochlorperazine
- Risperidone

Antimicrobial, antifungal and antimalarial drugs
- Chloroquine
- Clarithromycin
- Co-trimoxazole (trimethoprim–sulfamethoxazole)
- Erythromycin
- Ketoconazole
- Quinine

Antihistaminic drugs
- Fexofenadine

Others
- Alcohol
- Tacrolimus
- Tamoxifen

Prolonged QT interval due to amiodarone

Note
- Sinus rhythm
- First degree block
- Normal QRS complexes
- QT interval 600 ms
- Widespread T wave inversion

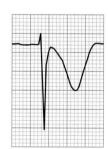

Long QT interval and inverted T wave in lead V_3

Fig. 7.21

Quinidine toxicity

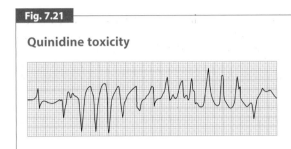

Note
- A single sinus beat is followed by a run of torsade de pointes ventricular tachycardia
- Although quinidine has now been withdrawn as a prescribable drug, alternative drugs, such as flecainide, might have the same effect

Fig. 7.22

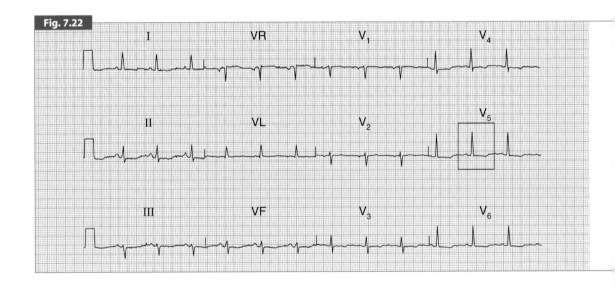

'Quinidine syncope' was recognized years before its mechanism was understood, and the ECG in Figure 7.21 is from a patient who developed TdP VT while being treated with quinidine.

Any of the drugs listed in Box 7.4 should be discontinued if the corrected QT interval exceeds 500 ms, or if the patient has symptoms suggesting an arrhythmia. It is prudent not to use drugs known to prolong the QT interval in patients with heart disease, and combinations of these drugs (e.g. erythromycin and ketoconazole) must definitely be avoided.

The appearance of T wave changes as, for example, in the patient needing lithium treatment whose ECG is shown in Figure 7.22, is not necessarily an indication to discontinue treatment.

Lithium treatment
Note
- Sinus rhythm
- Normal axis
- Normal QRS complexes
- Normal QT interval
- Widespread T wave inversion

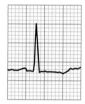

Inverted T wave in lead V₅

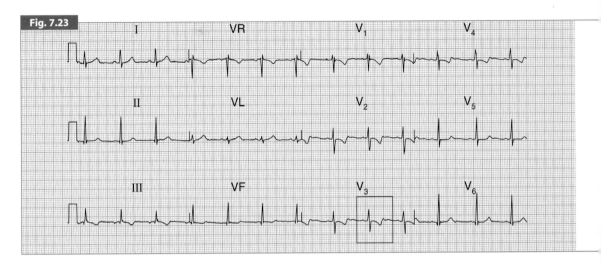

Fig. 7.23

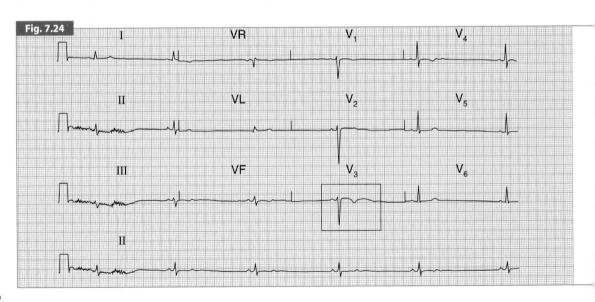

Fig. 7.24

Trauma

Note
- Sinus rhythm
- Normal axis
- Partial right bundle branch block pattern
- Anterior T wave inversion

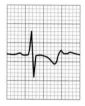

Inverted T wave in lead V₃

Anorexia nervosa

Note
- Sinus rhythm at 32/min
- Artefacts in leads II–III
- Normal axis
- Normal QRS complexes
- T wave inversion and U waves in anterior chest leads

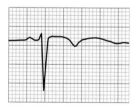

Inverted T wave and U wave in lead V₃

OTHER CAUSES OF AN ABNORMAL ECG

TRAUMA

Myocardial damage can be caused by chest injuries, either penetrating (e.g. stab wound) or closed (usually due to a steering wheel or seat belt). Direct trauma to the front of the heart can lead to occlusion of the left anterior descending coronary artery, and so to an ECG resembling that of an acute anterior myocardial infarction. However, seat belt injuries are more usually associated with myocardial contusion, as was the case in a young woman whose ECG is shown in Figure 7.23.

METABOLIC DISEASES

Most metabolic diseases, e.g. Addison's disease, are associated with nonspecific ST segment or T wave changes. There may be no apparent abnormality in the serum electrolytes. The ECG in Figure 7.24 is from a young girl with severe anorexia nervosa: her serum electrolytes and thyroid function were perfectly normal – the ECG changes presumably reflect an intracellular electrolyte abnormality.

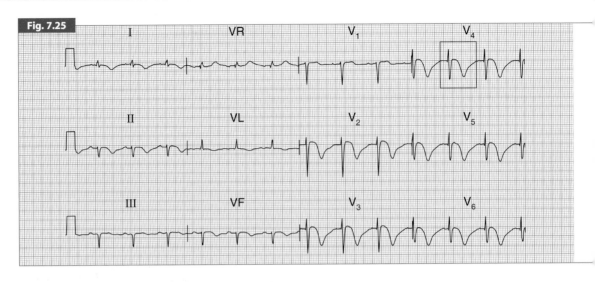

Fig. 7.25

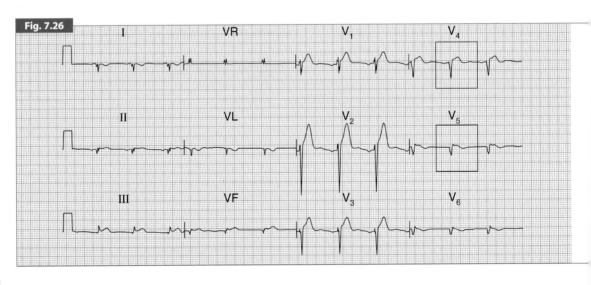

Fig. 7.26

Subarachnoid haemorrhage

Note

- Sinus rhythm
- Left axis deviation
- QT interval 600 ms
- Widespread T wave inversion

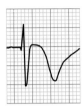

Long QT interval and inverted T wave in lead V₄

CEREBROVASCULAR ACCIDENTS

The association of a cerebrovascular accident and ECG abnormalities always suggests that the neurological problem is secondary to a cerebral embolus, which can arise in the heart because of an arrhythmia or a left ventricular thrombus.

Sudden intracerebral events, particularly subarachnoid haemorrhage, can cause widespread T wave inversion. The ECG in Figure 7.25 is from a patient with subarachnoid haemorrhage.

MUSCLE DISEASE

Many of the neuromuscular disorders are associated with a cardiomyopathy. The ECG in Figure 7.26 is from a young man with no cardiovascular symptoms and a clinically normal heart, who had Friedreich's ataxia.

Friedreich's ataxia

Note

- Sinus rhythm
- Right axis deviation
- Widespread T wave abnormality
- Appearances could suggest anterolateral ischaemia

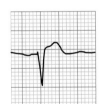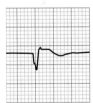

Changes in leads V₄ and V₅ suggesting an anterior infarction

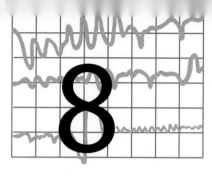

8 Conclusions: four steps to making the most of the ECG

Description	346
Interpretation	347
Diagnosis	348
Treatment	348
Conclusion	349

The theme of this book has been that the ECG is just one way of helping with the management of patients. The ECG is not an end in itself, and must always be seen in the context of the patient from whom it was recorded. To make the most of an ECG you need to think in four steps:

1. Describe it.
2. Interpret it.
3. See how it helps with the diagnosis.
4. Ask how it helps with treatment.

DESCRIPTION

An ECG can be described by anyone with the most basic knowledge, and an accurate description is needed as a basis for the later steps. The description starts with the heart rate and regularity, as measured by the intervals between the QRS complexes. The P waves must be identified; and if there are none, a clear statement of their absence is necessary. The relationship of the P waves to the QRS complexes is the next logical step, and the PR interval must be measured. The shape of the P wave needs to be recorded if it is abnormally peaked or bifid.

The QRS complexes need to be described in terms of their width and height, and also their shape: whether Q waves are present; whether there is more than one R wave in the QRS complex; and whether there are S waves in the leads where they would be expected. If there are Q waves, are they small and narrow, and are they only seen in the lateral leads, where they may be due to septal depolarization? If there are pathological Q waves, in which leads are they present and do they suggest a possible inferior or anterior myocardial infarction? The cardiac axis should be defined.

Elevation or depression of the ST segment must be noted. If the ST segment is elevated, does it follow an S wave, so indicating high take-off? The T waves must be inspected in each lead, and while inversion in VR and V_1 is always normal, inversion in any other leads should be recorded. The QT interval should be measured, and if it appears long, should be corrected for heart rate.

All these features can be identified without any knowledge of the patient, or indeed much knowledge of cardiology. The description of an ECG is reasonably well done by the automatic 'interpretation' function built into most modern ECG recorders, but it is important to remember that these are far from perfect. Automatic recorders tend to over-interpret ECGs so that nothing of importance is missed, and their descriptions are not always totally accurate. They can be poor at identifying P waves and they often miss ST segment changes, and sometimes T wave inversion. Therefore, you should never depend solely on a description provided by the ECG recorder itself.

INTERPRETATION

Always establish the cardiac rhythm first, because it may influence your interpretation of the rest of the ECG. For example, ventricular tachycardia, with its broad QRS complexes, will prevent any further interpretation – as will the broad complexes of complete heart block. The rhythm is established from the presence or absence of P waves and their relationship to the QRS complexes, from which arrhythmias and conduction defects can be accurately identified. On the whole, this part of ECG interpretation can be independent of the patient.

Otherwise, the accurate interpretation of an ECG should depend on a knowledge of the patient. If the ECG has been recorded from a healthy subject, or a patient with no clinical suggestion of cardiac disease, then it is essential to remember the range of normality of the ECG. First degree block, and supraventricular or ventricular extrasystoles, are commonly seen in healthy people. P waves can be bifid in healthy people; right axis deviation can be normal in tall thin people; and minor degrees of apparent left axis deviation with a narrow QRS complex can occur in fat people and in pregnancy. An RSR[1] pattern with a normal QRS complex duration in lead V_1 is perfectly normal, and in some perfectly normal people there can be a small dominant R wave in lead V_1. Tall QRS complexes are frequently seen in healthy young people, and do not in themselves indicate left ventricular hypertrophy. Septal Q waves may be present in leads VL and V_5–V_6. Inverted T waves in the anterior chest leads can be normal in black people, while in white people they may be due to hypertrophic cardiomyopathy. Peaked T waves are often of no significance at all, though they can be due to hyperkalaemia.

In a patient with chest pain, however, the interpretation of the same ECG abnormalities can be quite different. T wave inversion in the anterior chest leads may indicate an NSTEMI. Left bundle branch block may be the result of an old or new infarction. A change of cardiac axis to the right may be due to a pulmonary embolism. A dominant R wave in lead V_1 might be due to a posterior myocardial infarction.

In a patient with breathlessness, right axis deviation, a dominant R wave in lead V_1 or T wave inversion in leads V_1–V_3 may indicate multiple pulmonary emboli or idiopathic pulmonary hypertension. A deep S wave in lead V_6 may be due to chronic lung disease or to a pulmonary embolus. In patients complaining of attacks of dizziness, a finding such as first degree block, of little significance in a healthy subject, might indicate transient episodes of higher degrees of block causing a symptomatic bradycardia. A prolonged QT interval might point to episodes of torsade de pointes ventricular tachycardia.

Any described abnormality in an ECG must therefore be interpreted in the context of a knowledge of the patient's condition; otherwise, ECG changes will support a less focused differential diagnosis.

DIAGNOSIS

The ECG is essential for the diagnosis of problems involving rhythm and conduction, in which the interpretation and the diagnosis are clearly strongly linked. But it is necessary to remember that the identification of a specific arrhythmia does not complete the diagnosis, which should include the cause of the arrhythmia. For example, the cause of atrial fibrillation may be ischaemic or rheumatic heart disease, or alcoholism, or thyrotoxicosis, or a cardiomyopathy, and so on. Heart block may be due to idiopathic His bundle fibrosis, but it also raises the possibility of ischaemic or hypertensive heart disease. Left bundle branch block may be due to aortic stenosis, and right bundle branch block may be associated with an atrial septal defect.

ECG appearances that suggest faults in the recording technique may sometimes point to a clinical diagnosis. For example, artefacts due to movement may suggest a neurological disorder such as Parkinson's disease. Low-voltage QRS complexes may be due not to poor standardization but to obesity, emphysema, myxoedema or a pericardial effusion.

An ECG cannot diagnose the presence of heart failure, though with a totally normal ECG, heart failure is unlikely. The ECG may, however, help in diagnosing the cause of heart failure, which is often the key to treatment – atrial fibrillation, ventricular hypertrophy or left bundle branch block may suggest valve disease, or there may be evidence of an old myocardial infarction. Similarly, the ECG is not a good way of identifying electrolyte abnormalities, but flat T waves, U waves, and long QT intervals should at least suggest the possibility that there may be an electrolyte problem. A long QT interval, on the other hand, may be due to one of the congenital syndromes or to one of a wide variety of drugs.

The accurate identification of an ECG abnormality is thus only part of the diagnostic process: we still need to determine the underlying cause. The ECG often points the way to appropriate further investigations, such as chest X-rays, echocardiography, blood tests for electrolyte abnormalities, or cardiac catheterization, and the ECG is simply part of the diagnostic process.

TREATMENT

The ECG is obviously paramount in determining the treatment of an arrhythmia or conduction defects. It is also crucial for the proper use of acute interventions in both STEMIs and NSTEMIs. But its limitations must also be understood: in particular, it must be remembered that the ECG can be normal in the early stages of a myocardial infarction, and a normal, or near-normal, ECG is not an adequate reason for sending a patient with chest pain home from an A & E department.

Without an understanding of the ECG, devices such as pacemakers and implanted cardioverter defibrillators (ICDs) could not have been invented. These devices, and the techniques that use them, such as dual chamber pacing and cardiac resynchronization therapy, are the province of the specialist. But as the devices and techniques become increasingly prevalent, they will be encountered more and more by general practitioners and specialists in non-cardiac disciplines. For example, patients with these devices tend to be elderly, and it is the elderly who most frequently experience multiple medical problems – so non-cardiac specialists are bound to come across patients who have problems, but who also have a modern electrical device that is working perfectly normally.

CONCLUSION

The ECG is easy to describe and interpret, but it is often more difficult to appreciate the range of normality, and to remember that a full diagnosis encompasses the cause of any abnormality that may have been identified. The ECG is an essential part of the overall diagnostic process in a wide variety of patients, and in some it influences treatment. The most important thing to remember is that diagnosis and management depend on a full consideration of the individual patient, not just of the ECG.

NOW TEST YOURSELF

150 ECG Problems, a companion to this volume, gives 150 clinical scenarios with full related ECGs, and poses questions about ECG interpretation and the diagnosis and management of patients.

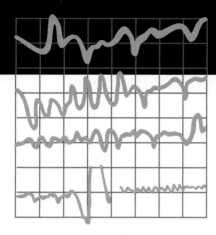

Index

Note: Page numbers in **bold** refer to figures and tables.
Abbreviations used in subentries: LBBB, left bundle branch block; RBBB, right bundle branch block;
RVOT-VT, right ventricular outflow tract ventricular tachycardia; WPW syndrome, Wolff–Parkinson–White syndrome.

A

'A' wave 184, **185**, **186**
AAI pacing *see* right atrial pacemakers
     (AAI)
ablation therapy *see* catheter ablation
abnormal ECG
     artefacts causing 316–317, 348
     asymptomatic, treatment 56
     congenital heart disease 320–327
     electrolyte abnormalities 331–335
     in healthy people 54–56
          actions to take 54
          ECG variations seen 55
          frequency 54
          prognosis 54–55
     management 56
     metabolic diseases **342–343**, 343
     muscle disease **344–345**, 345
     muscle movement causing 316–317, **317**
     subarachnoid haemorrhage **344–345**, 345
     systemic diseases 327, 329
     trauma **342–343**, 343
accelerated idionodal rhythm **48–49**, 49,
     102, **103**, **104**
     Lown–Ganong–Levine syndrome *vs* 72

accelerated idioventricular rhythm **28–29**,
     29, 102, **103**
accessory pathways 69, 72, 106, 147–149
     ablation 157, 158, **159**
     'bystander' 149
     drugs slowing conduction 155
     endocardial ECG and ablation 157, **159**
acute coronary syndrome 212, 264
acute rheumatic fever 289
Addison's disease 343
adenosine 154, 155
adrenaline 164
AH interval 184, **185**
alcoholism, atrial fibrillation 56
ambulatory ECG recording (Holter) 64,
     96–100
     monitoring devices **98–99**
amiodarone
     prolonged QT interval due to 77, **78–79**,
          154–155, 338, **338–339**
     torsade de pointes ventricular tachycardia
          due to 146, 338
     in ventricular tachycardia 150, 154–155
aneurysm, left ventricular 225
angina
     atypical 265, **266**

chest pain differential diagnosis 211
     diagnosis, NICE guidelines 265, 267
     ECG 212
     prevalence 265, **266**
     Prinzmetal's 'variant' **246**, 247
     stable 41, 213
     unstable 213
     see also chest pain
angiography
     left coronary artery 219
     right coronary artery 215
anorexia nervosa **342–343**, 343
anti-tachycardia pacing, ICD 167
antiarrhythmic drugs 150
     prolonged QT interval due to 338, 339
     torsade de pointes ventricular tachycardia
          due to 338, 339, 341
anticoagulation, atrial flutter/fibrillation 154
antidromic reciprocating tachycardia 106,
     107, **108**, 147
anxiety
     breathlessness 287
     sinus tachycardia 3, 113, 291
     T wave inversion 45
aortic dissection 210, 251
aortic regurgitation 209, 288

aortic stenosis 251, 288, **321**
 LBBB with **296–297**, 297
 left ventricular hypertrophy with
  322–323, 323
 severe, left ventricular hypertrophy with
  297, **298–299**
 syncope 64, **64–65**
arrhythmia 59
 ambulatory ECG recordings 150
 arterial pulse and **103**
 breathlessness and 289, 291
 diagnosis/investigations 150
 digoxin causing 335, 337
 electrophysiology 102
 exercise precipitating 150
 exercise test discontinuation 271
 in healthy people, ambulatory ECGs
  150
 heart rates associated **103**
 management 150, 164
  ablation 158
  non-shockable rhythms 164
  shockable rhythms 164
 precipitation 150
 prognosis 55
 syncope due to **61**
 see also individual arrhythmias
artefacts in ECG recordings 316–317, 348
asystole 60, **62–63**
 management 164
atenolol 154, 155
athletes
 left axis deviation **50–51**
 normal ECG 48–49, **50–51**
  rhythm and ECG pattern variations
   48–49
 PR interval 13, **48–49**, 49
 septal Q wave **50–51**
 sinus bradycardia 5
 sinus tachycardia 113
 T wave inversion in VL **50–51**
 U wave **50–51**
atrial extrasystoles 7, **114–115**, 115,
  226–227
atrial fibrillation **124–125**, 125, 176,
  178–179, 348
 alcoholism 56
 anterior ischaemia with 243, **244–245**
 asymptomatic, treatment 56

causes 116, 125
complete heart block with 176, **178**
conversion to sinus rhythm 154
digoxin effect **280–281**, **334–335**, 335,
  336
 on exercise **280–281**
 ischaemia and 257, **262–263**
 prophylactic 154
 at rest **280–281**
healthy people with abnormal ECG,
  prevalence 54
in hyperkalaemia **330–331**
in hypokalaemia **334–335**
inferior infarction with **140–141**, 141
investigations 56, **57**
irregular broad complex tachycardia
  126–127, **128–129**, 145, 147–149
irregular narrow complex tachycardia
  116, 117, **124–125**
LBBB with 127, **128–129**, **130–131**
in malignancy **328–329**, 329
management 56, 152, 154–155
 catheter ablation 158, **161**
 digoxin control of ventricular rate 335
 pacing 189, 195
in mitral stenosis 69, 288, 293
paroxysmal 69, 154
 prevention 154–155
permanent 154
persistent 154
prognosis 55
pulmonary embolism 247, **250–251**,
  310–311, 311
RBBB with **134–135**, 135
slow ventricular rate 170, 176
syncope 170
in thyroid disease 56, **326–327**, 327
uncontrolled 290–291, **290–291**
WPW syndrome with 73, **148–149**, 149,
  155
atrial flutter 109, 117, **118–119**, 176,
  176–177, **318–319**
1:1 conduction with 117, **120–121**
2:1 block with 117, **118–119**
4:1 block with 117, **120–121**
hypothermia 317, **318–319**
isthmus-dependent 109
management 154–155
 cardioversion 154–155

carotid sinus pressure 152, **153**
catheter ablation 158, **160**
intermittent VVI pacing 191, **194–195**
slow ventricular rate 176
variable block with 176, **176–177**
atrial pacing 197, **198–199**, 199, 201
 see also right atrial pacemakers (AAI)
atrial septal defect **321**
 RBBB with **326–327**, 327
atrial tachycardia 107, **110–111**, 111,
  116–117, 117
 2:1 block with 117
 carotid sinus pressure 152
 management 154
 palpitations and syncope **116–117**, 117
atrial tracking 199, **200–201**
atrioventricular block 179–186
 causes 184
 endocardial ECGs 184–186
 see also complete (third degree) block;
  first degree block; second degree
  block
atrioventricular nodal escape 175, **176**
atrioventricular nodal re-entry tachycardia
  (AVNRT) 109, **110**, **111**, 117,
  122–123, 123
 alternative names 109, 117
 bundle branch block with **126**
 carotid sinus pressure 152, **153**
 focal 102
 management 154
  ablation 158
 RBBB with 135, **136–137**
atrioventricular nodal reciprocating
  tachycardia 109
 see also atrioventricular nodal re-entry
  tachycardia (AVNRT)
atrioventricular node, ablation 158
atrioventricular re-entry tachycardia (AVRT)
  106–107, **107**
atrium
 automatic depolarization frequencies
  82–83
 silent 171, **174**
atropine 187
automaticity 82
 enhanced 102–105
  re-entry differentiation 111
 rhythms resulting from 82

Index

B

Bazett's formula 48
bicycle ergometer 270
bifascicular block 89, **90–91**
  prognosis 55
'bivent' *see* biventricular pacing
biventricular hypertrophy 288, **321**
  congenital heart disease **321**
biventricular pacemaker **207**
  chest X-ray **313**
biventricular pacing 165, 207, 312–313
  ECG appearance 313, **314–315**
  'obligate'/continuous 312
  see also cardiac resynchronization therapy
    (CRT)
black people, normal ECG 39, **42–43**
  T wave inversion 39, **42–43**, 252, 307,
    347
blood flow obstruction, syncope due to **61**
blood pressure, exercise testing 271
bradycardia 169–207
  ECG in **170–171**
  management 187–207
  mechanisms 169–186
    atrial fibrillation/flutter 176–178
    AV block 179–186
    sick sinus syndrome *see* sick sinus
      syndrome
  palpitations/syncope symptoms 82–95,
    171
    ECG between attacks 82–95
  syncope due to **61**, 169
bradycardia–tachycardia syndrome 171, **175**
breathlessness 287–312
  anxiety-induced sinus tachycardia 291
  atrial septal defect 327
  causes 287, 288, 289
  chronic lung disease 307, **310–311**
  disorders affecting left side of heart
    293–302
    left atrial hypertrophy **292–293**, 293
  disorders affecting right side of heart
    303–311
    right atrial hypertrophy **304–305**, 305
    right ventricular hypertrophy 305–311,
      306–307, **308–309**
  ECG value 289
  history and examination 287–289

palpitations with 291
pulmonary embolism **310–311**, 311
rhythm problems 291
broad complex tachycardia **76**, 107,
  126–143, 347
  differentiation 145
  ECG analysis 127
  irregular 107, 126, 127
    atrial fibrillation in 126, 127, **128–129**,
      145, 147–149
  in myocardial infarction 127
  P waves 126, 127
  polymorphic 147–149
  QRS complex 131, 135
    duration 126, 127
  RVOT-VT **104–105**
  supraventricular 126
  types 126–127
  uncertain origin 135, **136–137**
  ventricular 126
  ventricular or supraventricular? 135,
    136–137, **138–139**, 139
  WPW syndrome associated 126,
    147–149, **148–149**
  see also ventricular tachycardia
Bruce protocol 270, **270**
Brugada syndrome **80–81**, 81
bundle branch block
  healthy people 25, 54–55
  junctional tachycardia with **126**
  left *see* left bundle branch block (LBBB)
  right *see* right bundle branch block
    (RBBB)
bundle of Kent 69, 106
'bystander' pathway 149

C

calcium abnormalities 330, **331**, 335
calcium scoring, CT 267, **268–269**
calibration, ECG 25
capture beat 127, 142, **142–143**, 145
cardiac arrest 162–167
cardiac axis 15
  ECG description 347
  ECG interpretation 347
  left axis deviation *see* left axis deviation
  'leftward' limit of normality **16–17**
  normal variations 54–55

right axis deviation *see* right axis
    deviation
  'rightward' limit of normality **14–15**, 15
cardiac electrophysiology *see*
    electrophysiology (cardiac)
cardiac memo **98–99**
cardiac resynchronization therapy (CRT)
    207, 312–313
  ECG appearance 313, **314–315**
  indications 312–313
  see also biventricular pacing
cardiac rhythm 347
  abnormalities due to re-entry 105–111
  normal 2, **2**, 54–55
cardiac Syndrome X 277
cardiomyopathy
  congestive 289, 337
  hypertrophic *see* hypertrophic
    cardiomyopathy
cardiopulmonary resuscitation (CPR) 164
cardioversion 150
  atrial fibrillation 154–155
  atrial flutter 117, **118–119**
  atrioventricular nodal re-entry
    tachycardia **122–123**, 123
  ventricular tachycardia **138–139**, 139
carotid sinus hypersensitivity **61**, 150, **151**
carotid sinus pressure (CSP) 150, **151**
  atrial flutter 152, **153**
  atrial tachycardia 152
  junctional tachycardia 123, 152, **153**
  sinus rhythm 152, **153**
  sinus tachycardia 113
  tachycardia management 152
catheter ablation (radiofrequency ablation
    mediated by) 102, 157, 158
  arrhythmias amenable to 156–158
  atrial fibrillation 158, **161**
  atrial flutter 158, **160**
  AV node 158
  electrophysiological mapping and 155,
    157
  left-sided accessory pathways 157, **159**
  paroxysmal atrial fibrillation 155
  pathways (AVNRE and WPW syndrome)
    158
  ventricular tachycardia 162
catheters, transvenous, fluoroscopic image
    156, **156**

cerebrovascular accidents **344–345**, 345
chest pain 209–286
  acute 210
    investigations 264–265
    management 264, 285
    suggestive of myocardial infarction 264
  anginal 265, **266**
  atypical 211
  causes 209
  chronic 211, 265
    causes 209
    investigations 265, **268–269**
    management 285–286
  ECG interpretation 264, 347
  ECG pitfalls 252–263
    false negatives/positives 252
    R wave changes **254–255**, 255,
      256–257
    ST segment and T wave changes
      256–257, **258–259**, **260–261**,
      262–263
    summary **253**
  exercise testing see exercise testing
  history and examination 209–211
  investigations 264–265
  left ventricular hypertrophy 251
  management 264, 285–286
  non-anginal 265, **266**
  pericarditis 251
  pulmonary embolism 209, 210
  recurrent, causes 209
  ST segment depression and 241, 243
  of unknown cause 211, 213
chest X-rays 264
  biventricular pacemaker **313**
  chest pain 264
  dual chamber pacemaker **198**
  fractured pacing lead 202, **203**
  ICD devices **166**, 167
  pacemaker assessment 187
  right atrial pacemakers **196**
  right atrial/ventricular lead displacement
    202, **202**
  right ventricular pacemaker **190**
  single chamber ICD **166**
children, normal ECG 52–53, 320
chronic lung disease 307, **310–311**
chronic obstructive pulmonary disease
    (COPD) 303

ECG feature summary 303
  right ventricular and right atrial
    hypertrophy **304–305**, 305
'circus movement' 106
clockwise rotation 21, **304–305**
  right ventricular hypertrophy 235, 305
complete (third degree) block 83, 89, 179,
    180–181
  atrial fibrillation with 176, **178**
  causes 184
  prognosis 54
  Stokes–Adams attack 179, **182–183**
  syncope due to 170
  VVI pacing **194–195**, 195
concordance, QRS complexes 127, 131,
    132–133, **134–135**, 135
conduction
  abnormalities, combinations 89–95
  anterograde (normal) 69, 105, **107**, 123
  delay **107**
  normal 69, 105, **107**, 123
  re-entry 69, 105, **105**, 106, **107**
  retrograde 83, 106
conduction defects 82–83
  healthy people with abnormal ECG 54–55
  prognosis 54–55
  see also heart block
congenital heart disease 320–327
  ECG appearance summary **321**
congenital long QT syndrome 76, **76–77**
cor pulmonale 289
coronary artery disease (CAD) 265
  exercise testing 273, 277
  left ventricular hypertrophy with 299,
    300–301
  NICE guidelines 267
  prevalence 265, **266**
coronary spasm 247
counterclockwise rotation 21
creatine kinase, CK-MB 212, 264
CRTD (cardiac resynchronization therapy
    defibrillator) 165, **207**, 313

D

defibrillation 164
  CRT device **207**, 313
  see also implanted cardioverter
    defibrillator (ICD) devices

delta wave 69
  WPW syndrome type A 69, **70–71**,
    72–73, 73, **108–109**, **148–149**,
    255, **256–257**
  WPW syndrome type B **74–75**, 256,
    258–259, **302–303**
depolarization 69, 82–83, 191
  atrial 82–83
  circular wave 69
  endocardial ECG 184
  late 105
  normal 69, 82–83
  pacemaker action 188
  reversed direction 105
  septal Q wave 29
  spontaneous (automaticity) 82–83
  WPW syndrome 69
  see also automaticity; conduction
dextrocardia **10–11**
  leads reversed 7, **10–11**
  P wave 7, **10–11**
digoxin 257, **262–263**, 335–337
  arrhythmias due to 335, 337
  atrial fibrillation/flutter 154, 335, **336**,
    336–337
  ECG diagnostic pitfalls **253**
  effects on ECG **334–335**, 335
    summary 337
  enhanced automaticity and 102
  exercise testing and 277, **280–281**
  ischaemia and 257, **262–263**
  ST segment depression 31, 257, **262–263**
    downward-sloping **253**, 257, **262–263**,
      334–335, **336–337**
  T wave inversion 257, **262–263**
  toxicity 117, 335, **336**, **336–337**, 337
    symptoms 335, 337
dizziness 60
  ECG interpretation 347–348
  exercise testing discontinuation 271
  sick sinus syndrome 171
  see also syncope
drugs
  effect on ECG 335–341
    see also digoxin
  prolonged QT interval 77, 144, 146,
    146–147, 338
    amiodarone 77, **78–79**, 79, 155, 338,
      338–339

353

torsade de pointes ventricular tachycardia
    due to 338, 339, **340**, 341
dual chamber pacemakers (DDD) 165, 188,
    189, 199–202, **207**
    atrial pacing with ventricular tracking
        201
    atrial tracking 199, **200–201**
    chest X-ray **198**, 199
    ECG appearance **198–199**, 199
    indications for 199
    magnet rate 206, **206**
    rate response (DDDR) 202
    specialist functions 202

E

Ebstein's anomaly **324–325**, 325
echocardiography 56, 150, 264, 265
    stress **268–269**
ectopic atrial rhythm 7, **8–9**
elderly
    thyroid disease **326–327**, 327
electrical alternans **328–329**, 329
electrolyte abnormalities
    diagnosis and ECG role 348
    effects on ECG 331–335
    prolonged QT syndrome due to 77
electromechanical dissociation (EMD) 164
electrophysiology (cardiac) 102, 155–161
    catheter ablation and 157
    complications 163
    endocardial ECGs 156, 157, 184
    indications 163
    mapping and catheter ablation **156**, 157
    purpose of studies 102
    scale of traces 157, **159**
    see also automaticity; re-entry, cardiac
        rhythm abnormalities due to
emphysema, QRS complex 348
endocardial ECGs 156, **156**, 157, 184
    in atrioventricular block 184–186
    left-sided accessory pathway ablation
        157, **159**
    real-time analysis 157
enhanced automaticity 102–105
    ablation therapy 157
    re-entry differentiation 111
escape beats **62–63**, 83
    junctional **5**, **82**, 83, **83**

ventricular **83**
escape rhythms 82–83, 169
'event recorders' 96
exercise
    arrhythmias precipitated by 150
    digoxin effect, in atrial fibrillation 277,
        280–281
    ischaemia induced by 271, **272–273**, 277,
        278–279
    ST segment elevation induced by
        274–275, 275
    ventricular extrasystoles induced by 282,
        284
    ventricular fibrillation induced by 282,
        284
    ventricular tachycardia induced by **151**
exercise testing 267, 270–284
    Bruce protocol 270, **270**
    chronic chest pain 267, **268–269**
    contraindications 283
    digoxin effect 277, **280–281**
    discontinuation reasons 271
    'false positive' 277, **280–281**
    information available from 267
    interpretation 271–272
    ischaemia **272–273**, 273
    normal **272–273**, 273, 277, **278–279**
    old myocardial infarction **274–275**, 275
    'positive' 271, 273, 277
    practical aspects 270–271
    pseudonormalization 275, **276–277**
    risks **282–283**, 283, **284**
    sensitivity/specificity 277
    ST segment depression **272–273**, 273,
        278–279
    ST segment elevation **274–275**, 275
    unreliable, conditions included 271
    ventricular extrasystole development 282,
        284
    ventricular fibrillation development 282,
        284
extrasystoles 59, 102, 106, 115
    atrial 7, **114–115**, 115, **226–227**
    enhanced automaticity causing 102
    healthy people 7, **7**, 96
    junctional 7, **114–115**, 115
    management 152
    palpitations due to 152
    symptoms due to 115

F

fainting see Stokes–Adams attack; syncope
Fallot's tetralogy **321**
    right ventricular hypertrophy **324–325**,
        325
'false positives,' exercise testing 277,
        280–281
fascicular tachycardia 135, **136–137**
first degree block **84–85**, 179
    causes 184
    His bundle electrogram 184, **185**
    His electrogram 184, **185**
    LBBB with **88–89**
    left anterior hemiblock with **88–89**, 89
    left posterior hemiblock with **92–93**
    prevalence 54
    prognosis 54
    RBBB with 89, **90–91**, **174–175**, 175,
        182–183
    RBBB and left anterior hemiblock with
        89, **90–91**
flecainide 155
focal junctional tachycardia 102
Fridericia's correction 48
Friedreich's ataxia **344–345**, 345
fusion beat 127, 142, **142–143**, 145

G

glyceryl trinitrate 265, 285
glycoprotein IIb/IIIa inhibitor 285

H

'H' spike 184, **185**, **186**
haemoglobin, measurement 265
healthy people
    abnormal ECG see under abnormal ECG
    arrhythmias, ambulatory ECG recordings
        150
    normal ECG variants see normal ECG
heart block 179–186, 347, 348
    causes 179, 184
    first degree see first degree block
    second degree see second degree block
    third degree see complete (third degree)
        block
    trifascicular block 89, **92–93**

see also bifascicular block
heart failure 288
  cardiac resynchronization therapy 312
  diagnosis and ECG role 312
heart rate 2–5
  arrhythmias 103, **103**
  control 82
  exercise testing 271
    discontinuation indication 271
  infants/young children 52
  maximum, calculation 271
  QT interval correction for 48
  sinus or paroxysmal tachycardia 59
  types of arrhythmia associated 103
herpes zoster, pain 210
His bundle
  endocardial ECG 184, **185**
  fibrosis 348
  orthodromic tachycardia 106
  re-entry circuit involving 69, 123
  re-entry tachycardia and 106
  slow conduction through 176
  in trifascicular block 89
His bundle electrogram
  first degree block 184, **185**
  normal 184, **185**
  second degree block 184, **186**
    2:1 block 184, **186**
Holter monitor **98–99**
HV interval 184, **185**
hypercalcaemia 330, 335
hyperkalaemia **330–331**, 331, **332–333**, 333
  peaked T wave 45
hypertrophic cardiomyopathy **68–69**, 299, **300–301**
  ECG diagnostic pitfalls **253**
  ECG features **68–69**, 289
  MR image **68**
  syncope due to **61**, 67, **68–69**, 69
hyperventilation 45
hypocalcaemia 330, 335
hypokalaemia 47, 330, **334–335**, 335
hypothermia 317, **318–319**
  atrial flutter 317, **318–319**

I

ICD see implanted cardioverter defibrillator
  (ICD) devices

idionodal rhythm, accelerated see
  accelerated idionodal rhythm
idioventricular rhythm, accelerated **28–29**, 29, 102, **103**
implantable loop recorder **98–99**
implanted cardioverter defibrillator (ICD)
  devices 165–167, 348
  anti-tachycardia pacing **166**, 167
  biventricular pacing and 313
  chest X-ray **166**, 167
  defibrillator function 167
  dual chamber (DDD/ICD) 165, **207**
  ECG appearance 167
  indications 167, 313
  pacemaker function 165
  single chamber 165, **166**
  tachycardia control 167
  ventricular fibrillation **166**
infants, ECG 52, **52–53**, 320
inspiration, normal ECG during 37, **38**
interpretation, ECG 312–313
intracardiac recordings 157, 184
ischaemia 212–246, **240–241**, 241
  anterior **242–243**, 243
    atrial fibrillation with 243, **244–245**
    AV nodal re-entry tachycardia with 243, **244–245**
    inferior infarction and RBBB with 237, **238–239**
    RBBB with 237, **238–239**
  anterolateral **242–243**, 243
    Friedreich's ataxia suggestive of **344–345**
  diagnosis by exercise testing **272–273**, 273
  digoxin effect vs 257, **262–263**
  exercise-induced 271, **272–273**, 277, **278–279**
  investigations 56
  lateral **216–217**
  left ventricular hypertrophy vs 256, **260–261**, **298–299**, 299, **300–301**
  normal variant confusion 252
  pseudonormalization 275, **276–277**
  without myocardial infarction **240–241**, 241, 243
isoprenaline 187
ivabradine 285

J

J point 35, 214, 273
  depression during exercise 277
J wave 317, **318–319**
'junctional' cells 82–83
junctional escape beat **5**, **82**, 83
junctional escape rhythm **82**, 82–83, **83**
  hyperkalaemia **330–331**
  sustained 83
junctional extrasystoles 7, **114–115**, 115
junctional region, automatic depolarization
  frequencies 82–83
junctional tachycardia 109, 117
  see also atrioventricular nodal re-entry
    tachycardia (AVNRT)

L

left anterior hemiblock 85, **88–89**, 89, **302–303**
  lateral T wave changes 299, **302–303**
  left axis deviation in **88–89**, 89, 295
  in left ventricular hypertrophy 295
  prognosis 54–55
  RBBB and 89, **90–91**, **92–93**
  RBBB and first degree block with 89, **92–93**
  second degree (2:1) block with 89, **94–95**
  second degree (2:1) block and RBBB with 89, **94–95**
left atrial hypertrophy 7, **70–71**, **292–293**, 293
  left ventricular hypertrophy with **292–293**, 293
  mitral stenosis 69
left axis deviation 15, 85, **86–87**, 89
  acute anterolateral infarction with **222–223**, **224–225**, 225
  anterior NSTEMI **240–241**, 241
  athletes **50–51**
  bifascicular block **90–91**
  congenital heart disease **321**
  left anterior hemiblock **88–89**, 89, **300–301**
  left ventricular hypertrophy 295
  normal ECG 15, 55, 85, 89, 347
  pregnancy 15, 55

355

prevalence 54
ventricular tachycardia, in infarction 131, **132–133**
left bundle branch block (LBBB) **66–67**, 235, 348
aortic stenosis with **296–297**, 297
cardiac resynchronization therapy 312
causes 235, 347
first degree block with **88–89**, 89
healthy people with abnormal ECG 54–55, 56
investigations 56, **57**
myocardial infarction with **234–235**, 235
prevalence 54
prognosis 54–55
left coronary artery, normal/occluded **219**, **221**, 231
left main coronary artery **219**, **221**
narrowing 257
left posterior hemiblock 89, **92–93**
left ventricle, contraction, in LBBB 312
left ventricular aneurysm 225
left ventricular hypertrophy 251, **252–253**, **260–261**, **294–295**, 295, **296–297**, 297
aortic dissection and 251
aortic stenosis **322–323**, 323
severe aortic stenosis with 297, **298–299**
syncope due to 64, **64–65**
causes 295, 297
congenital heart disease 320, **321**, **322–323**
ECG features 295
ECG pitfalls **253**, 256
ECGs/conditions mimicking 256, 299–303
in infants/young children 52, 320, **321**
ischaemia *vs* **298–299**, 299, **300–301**
lateral ischaemia *vs* 256, **260–261**
left atrial hypertrophy with **292–293**, 293
voltage criteria **294–295**, 295, 297
left ventricular strain 297
lidocaine (lignocaine), ventricular tachycardia 155
lithium treatment, ECG in **340–341**, 341
long QT syndrome 76–77
congenital 76, **76–77**, **78–79**
management 155

drug toxicity *see* drugs, prolonged QT interval
ECG interpretation pitfall and 256, **258–259**
genetic abnormalities 76
management 155
syncope due to **61**
loop recorder **98–99**
Lown–Ganong–Levine syndrome 72, **74–75**
re-entry pathway **105**
lung disease
chronic, persistent S wave 307, **310–311**
right ventricular hypertrophy *vs* 307
see also chronic obstructive pulmonary disease (COPD)

M

'macro re-entrant' circuits 109
magnesium
serum levels, abnormal **331**, 335
therapeutic 155
magnet rate, pacemakers 206, **206**
mapping/ablation catheter 157
mediastinal shift 21, **22–23**
metabolic diseases, abnormal ECG **342–343**, 343
metabolic equivalents (METs) 270
workloads expressed in 270
mitral regurgitation 288
mitral stenosis 69, 288, 293
atrial fibrillation 69, 288, 293
left atrial hypertrophy 69
pulmonary hypertension and **292–293**, 293
mitral valve prolapse 288
muscle disease **344–345**, 345
muscle movement, abnormal 316–317, **317**
myocardial infarction
acute chest pain suggestive of **253**
anterior 217, **218–219**, 225
acute 213
acute, and old inferior infarction 231, **232–233**
NSTEMI **240–241**, 241
old 213, **224–225**, 225
old, acute inferior infarction with **230–231**, 231
old, exercise testing **274–275**, 275

old inferior infarction with 231, **232–233**
poor R wave progression **230–231**, 231
RBBB with **236–237**, 237
V_2–V_5 leads 217, **218–219**
anterolateral 217, 243
acute 217, **222–223**, 225
acute, with left axis deviation 217, **222–223**
age unknown **224–225**, 225
old **224–225**, 225
old, NSTEMI 257, **260–261**
broad complex tachycardia 126–127, 135
CABG-related 213
definition 212
diagnosis/ECG 212, **254**, 264
ECG changes, sequence of features, in STEMI 213, **214–215**, 264
ECG pitfalls **252**, **253**
elevated ST segment 31
false positives/negatives **253**
full thickness 241
hyperacute, peaked T wave **44–45**, 45
inferior 215
acute **214–215**, 215, **230–231**
anterior ischaemia with **230–231**, 231
anterior NSTEMI with 231, **232–233**
atrial fibrillation with **140–141**, 141
evolving 214, **214–215**, **216–217**
old **84–85**
old, acute anterior infarction with 231, **232–233**
old, anterior ischaemia with **240–241**, 241
RBBB and possible anterior ischaemia with 237, **238–239**
right ventricular infarction 228, **228–229**
ventricular tachycardia with **140–141**, 141
lateral 217
acute **220–221**
after 3 days 217, **222–223**
LBBB with **234–235**, 235
management 285–286
multiple **230–231**, 231, **232–233**
non-Q wave *see* NSTEMI
nonspecific ST segment/T wave changes **210–211**

NSTEMI (non-ST segment elevation) *see* NSTEMI
PCI-related 213
posterior 226–227, **226–227**
  dominant R wave in lead V₁ **226–227**, 227, 307
  old **254–255**, 255
prior, criteria for 213
secondary to ischaemia 213
serial ECG recordings 225
STEMI (ST segment elevation) *see* STEMI
subendocardial 241
temporary pacing 187
types 213
ventricular tachycardia 131, **132–133**
without ischaemia **240–241**, 241
myocardial perfusion scintigraphy **268–269**
myocarditis, ECG feature summary 289
myxoedema, QRS complex 348

N

narrow complex tachycardia 116, 117–125
  irregular, atrial fibrillation 116, 117, **124–125**
  types 116
  see also atrial fibrillation; atrial flutter; atrial tachycardia; atrioventricular nodal re-entry tachycardia (AVNRT)
NICE guidance
  angina diagnosis 265
  coronary artery disease diagnosis 267
nicorandil 285
non-Q wave infarction *see* NSTEMI
non-segment elevation myocardial infarction (NSTEMI) *see* NSTEMI
normal ECG 1–53, **8–9**, **12–13**, 13, **18–19**, 347
  in athletes 48–49, **50–51**
  in black people 39, **42–43**, 252, 347
  cardiac axis 54–55
    left axis deviation 15, 55, 85, 89, 347
    'leftward' limit of normality **16–17**
    right axis deviation 15, **16–17**, 55, 347
    'rightward' limit of normality **14–15**
  children 52–53, 320
  endocardial 184, **185**

exercise testing **272–273**, 273, 277, **278–279**
extrasystoles 7, **7**, 96
heart rate 2–5
  on inspiration 37, **38**
interpretation 347
left axis deviation 15, 55, 85, 89, 347
P wave 7–11
  inversion 7, **40–41**
  normal variations 54–55
  notched (bifid) 7, **12–13**, 293, 347
  peaked 7
partial RBBB pattern 25, **26–27**
PR interval **8–9**, **12–13**, 13
  athletes **48–49**, 49
Q wave **28–29**, 29, 252, 347
QRS complex **14–15**, 15, 117
  normal variants 55
  'splintered' 25
  width 25
QT interval 48, **78–79**
QTc 48
R wave **300–301**
  dominant wave in lead V₁ 21, **22–23**, 253, **254–255**, 255, 307, **308–309**
  size **16–17**, 19–25, **24–25**, 25
range of normality 54–55
right axis deviation 15, **16–17**, 55, **306**, 307, 347
right ventricular hypertrophy and 39, **253**
RS complexes 54–55
S wave
  dominant in lead V₄ **20–21**, 21
  size 15, **16–17**, 19–25, **24–25**, 25
ST segment 31–37
  depression 31, **34–35**
  elevation 31, **32–33**
  exercise testing **272–273**
  high take-off 31, **32–33**
  nonspecific depression 31, 35, **36–37**
  normal variations 31, **32–35**, **36–37**, 55
  upward-sloping **30–31**, 31
supraventricular extrasystoles **6–7**, 7, **7**, 55
T wave 37–47
  biphasic (V₃) **40–41**
  flattening **44–45**, 45

normal variants 39, 45, **54–55**
  peaked, normal ECG **12–13**, **44–45**, 45, **332–333**, 333
T wave inversion **36–37**, 37
  in black people 39, **42–43**, 252, 307, 347
  dominant R wave (V₁) with 307, **308–309**
  lead III 37, **38–39**, 39
  in VR **36–37**, 37
  transition point between V₂ and V₃ **20–21**, 21
U wave **46–47**, 47, 55
variants 54–55
  ischaemia *vs* 252, **253**
  summary 54–55
ventricular extrasystoles **6–7**, 7
voltage criteria and left ventricular hypertrophy **294–295**, 295, 297
NSTEMI 67, 213, **240–241**, 241, 256, 347
  acute inferior infarction with 231, **232–233**
  anterior **240–241**, 241
  hypertrophic cardiomyopathy *vs* 67
  management 285
  old anterolateral 257, **260–261**
  risk categories 285
  STEMI *vs* 241, 264

O

obesity 15
  QRS complex 347
oesophageal rupture, pain 210
orthodromic reciprocating tachycardia 106, **108**
orthopnoea 289
overdrive pacing 167
oxygen, rate of use, metabolic equivalents 270

P

P mitrale 293
P pulmonale 305
P wave 7, **8–13**, 127
  atrial flutter 117, **118–119**
  atrial tachycardia **116–117**, 117
  bifid (notched) 7, **64–65**, 293

357

Index

left atrial hypertrophy **70–71**, **292–293**, 293

mitral stenosis and pulmonary hypertension **292–293**, 293

normal ECG 7, **12–13**, 293, 347

broad complex tachycardia 126, 127

complete heart block **180–181**

dextrocardia 7, **10–11**

flattened/absent, hyperkalaemia **330–331**, 331

following QRS complex, junctional escape rhythm **82**, 83

inverted 7, **8–9**, **10–11**, **40–41**
  atrial tachycardia 107, **110–111**
  normal ECG 7, **40–41**

junctional escape rhythms **82–83**, 83

nodal rhythm overtaking, accelerated idionodal rhythm 102, **104**

normal variations 7–9, 12–13, **40–41**, 54–55

peaked 7
  normal people 7
  pulmonary embolism 247, **248–249**
  right atrial hypertrophy 7, 235, **304–305**, 305
  right atrial hypertrophy and RBBB in Ebstein's anomaly **324–325**
  right ventricular hypertrophy **306–307**

'sawtooth' 117, **118–119**

second degree block **87–88**
  left anterior hemiblock and **94–95**
  left anterior hemiblock and RBBB and **94–95**

supraventricular extrasystoles **114–115**, 115

pacemakers 187–207
  abnormal function 202–206
  'backup,' VVI 189, 191
  biventricular 207
  dual chamber *see* dual chamber pacemakers
  failed pacing capture 202, **204**
  failure 202
  functions 187
  ICD devices 165, 167
  indications **207**
  magnet rate 206, **206**
  nomenclature 188
  over-sensing or far-field sensing 203, **205**

right atrial *see* right atrial pacemakers (AAI)

right ventricular *see* right ventricular pacemakers (VVI)

single-chamber 188, **189**, **207**
  tachycardia mediated by 203, **205**
  types **189**, **207**
  under-sensing 203, **204**, **205**

pacing 187–207
  bipolar 188, **190–191**, 191
  description 188
  failed capture 202, **204**
  'overdrive' 167
  temporary, in acute myocardial infarction 187
  unipolar 188, 191, **192–193**

pacing lead 189, **191**
  atrial 199
  displacement 202, **202**

palpitations 58–64
  ambulatory ECG 96, **98–99**
  bradycardia causing 82–95, 171
    ECG between attacks 82–95
    escape rhythms 82–83
  causes 152
  clinical history and diagnosis 59–64, **61**
  diagnosis of cause 64
  ECG features, between attacks 64–95
  extrasystoles causing 152
  physical examination 64, 103
  tachycardias causing **59**, 69–81, 152
    atrial fibrillation 152
    Brugada syndrome 81
    long QT syndrome 76–77
    mitral stenosis 69
    paroxysmal tachycardia **59**
    pre-excitation and WPW syndromes 69–72
    sinus tachycardia **59**, 113, 152
    supraventricular tachycardia 152
    ventricular tachycardia 152
  thyroid disease 327

Parkinsonism 317, **317**

paroxysmal tachycardia 59
  diagnosis from symptoms 59, **59**

paroxysmal ventricular tachycardia 76, 155

partial RBBB pattern 25, **26–27**, **34–35**, **134–135**, 135, **292–293**
  trauma associated **342–343**

percutaneous coronary interventions (PCI) 285
  myocardial infarction related to 213

pericardial effusion
  malignant **328–329**, 329
  QRS complex 348

pericardial pain 209, 210

pericarditis 209, 212, **250–251**, 251
  causes 264

pneumothorax 165, 210, 264

post-ventricular atrial refractory period (PVARP) 203

postural hypotension **61**

potassium abnormalities 330, **331**, **332–333**, **334–335**

PR interval **12–13**, 13
  athletes 13, **48–49**, 49
  atrial tachycardia 107
  in ECG description 346
  normal **12–13**, 13, **48–49**
  prolonged
    first degree block **84–85**
    left posterior hemiblock **92–93**
    second degree block **84–85**, **180–181**
    trifascicular block **92–93**
  short
    atrial tachycardia 107
    Lown–Ganong–Levine syndrome 72, **74–75**
    WPW syndrome, type A **70–71**, **72–73**, **108–109**, **148–149**
    WPW syndrome, type B **74–75**, **302–303**
  variation, accelerated idionodal rhythm **48–49**, 49

pre-excitation syndromes 69, 106
  see also Lown–Ganong–Levine syndrome; Wolff–Parkinson–White (WPW) syndrome

pregnancy, ECG 15, 52, 347
  left axis deviation 15, 55
  right axis deviation 15
  ST segment depression 55
  ventricular extrasystoles 52, 54

Prinzmetal's 'variant' angina **246**, 247

prognosis, abnormal ECG 54

pseudonormalization 275, **276–277**

psychiatric drugs, prolonged QT interval due to 339

pulmonary embolism 209
    chest pain 209, 210, 265
    ECG 212, **246–247**, 247, **250–251**
    ECG feature summary 247, 303
    right axis deviation 247, **248–249**, **250–251**
    right ventricular hypertrophy and 307, 311
    T wave inversion 39, **246–247**, 247, **248–249**
pulmonary hypertension
    idiopathic 303
    mitral stenosis and **292–293**, 293
    thromboembolic 67, 247, 303
pulmonary stenosis **322–323**, 323
pulmonary vein, isolation by ablation 158, **161**
pulseless electrical activity (PEA) 164
    causes and management 164
pulseless ventricular tachycardia, management 164

Q

Q wave 29
    in ECG description 346–347
    myocardial infarction 213, 214
        acute anterior and old inferior infarctions 231, **232–233**
        acute inferior and old anterior **230–231**, 231
        acute inferior STEMI **214–215**
        acute inferior STEMI and anterior (NSTEMI) 231, **232–233**
        acute lateral STEMI **220–221**
        evolving inferior STEMI **216–217**
        inferior and right ventricular infarction 228, **228–229**
        inferior infarction and RBBB and anterior ischaemia 237, **238–239**
        lateral STEMI (3 days old) **222–223**
        old anterior infarction **274–275**, 275
        posterior infarction **226–227**, 227
    septal **28–29**, 29, 252, 347
        in athletes **50–51**
    small 29, **30–31**
        inferior infarction **140–141**
QRS complex **14–15**, 15, **15**

alternate large and small (electrical alternans) **328–329**, 329
broad
    VVI bipolar pacing and **190–191**, 191
broad complex tachycardia 126–127, 131, 135
    duration 126, 127
    cardiac axis and 15
    concordance 127, 131, **132–133**, **134–135**, 135
    extrasystoles 115
    healthy people **14–15**, 15, 117, 347
    LBBB pattern 127, **128–129**
        RVOT-VT **144–145**
        ventricular tachycardia **145**
    left ventricular hypertrophy **294–295**, 295
    myocardial infarction 131, 135
    narrow, supraventricular extrasystoles 115
    narrow complex tachycardias 117–125
    normal ECG **14–15**, 15, 117, 347
    normal variations 55
    RBBB pattern **134–135**, 135
        complete heart block **180–181**
        ventricular tachycardia **140–141**, **142–143**, 145
    slurred upstroke see delta wave
    small, in malignancy **328–329**, 329
    splintered 25
    tall 15, **260–261**
        healthy people 347
        left atrial and left ventricular hypertrophy **292–293**
    ventricular tachycardia 127, **130**, 131
    widened
        complete heart block **180–181**
        left axis deviation with (left anterior hemiblock) 85, **88–89**, 89
        ventricular extrasystoles 115
        ventricular tachycardia due to re-entry 109
        see also broad complex tachycardia
    width 126, 127
        normal variants 25
        RSR^{1}S^1 pattern 25, **26–27**
        see also RSR^1 pattern
    Wolff–Parkinson–White syndrome 69, **70–71**, **70–75**

'QS' complexes **132–133**
QT interval 48
    correction for heart rate (QT$_c$) 48, 77
    normal
        posterior infarct with **78–79**
        upper limit 48
    prolonged 76–77, **78–79**
        amiodarone causing 77, **78–79**, 79, 155, 338, **338–339**
        causes 76, 77
        drugs causing see drugs, prolonged QT interval
        hypocalcaemia 335
        hypokalemia 335
        subarachnoid haemorrhage **344–345**
        unexplained, with T wave abnormality 256, **258–259**
QT$_c$
    long QT syndrome 77
    normal ECG 48
    sudden death risk and 77
quinidine syncope 341

R

R on T phenomenon 115, **116**, **162–163**
    in healthy people 96
R wave 19–25
    dominant in lead V$_1$ 21, **22–23**, 255, **256–257**
    causes **306**, 307
    normal variant 21, **22–23**, 253, **254–255**, 255, 307, **308–309**
    old posterior infarction **254–255**, 255
    posterior infarction **226–227**, 227, 307
    pulmonary embolism 247
    pulmonary stenosis **322–323**
    right ventricular hypertrophy **66–67**, 255, 305, **306–307**
    right ventricular hypertrophy in Fallot's tetralogy **324–325**
    WPW type A **108–109**, 255, **256–257**
    ECG interpretation pitfalls and **254–255**, 255
    height 25
    normal **300–301**
    poor progression, anterior infarction **224–225**, 225, **230–231**, 231
S wave size balance 25

second peak **134–135**, 135, **136–137**
size, in chest leads **16–17**, **18–19**, 19–25,
    24–25
slurred upstroke (delta wave) **70–71**,
    72–73, **108–109**, 255, **256–257**
tall
    left ventricular hypertrophy **64–65**,
        252–253, **294–295**, 295
    WPW syndrome type B **300–301**
re-entry, cardiac rhythm abnormalities due
    to **105**, 105–111
    AVNRT *see* atrioventricular nodal
        re-entry tachycardia (AVNRT)
    enhanced automaticity differentiation
        111
    tachycardia 69
    ventricular tachycardia 109, **110**
re-entry pathway 69, 105, **105**, 106, **107**
    Lown–Ganong–Levine syndrome **105**
    WPW type A syndrome **105**
'reciprocating tachycardia' 106
repolarization 256
    delayed 76
'reverse tick' 335
rheumatic fever, acute 289
right atrial hypertrophy 7, **304–305**, 305
    congenital heart disease **321**, **324–325**,
        325
    Ebstein's anomaly **324–325**, 325
    peaked P wave 7, **304–305**, 305
    RBBB and **324–325**, 325
    right ventricular hypertrophy with 67,
        304–305, 305
right atrial pacemakers (AAI) **196–197**, 197
    chest X-ray **196**
    ECG appearance **196–197**, 197
    indications 197, **207**
    rate response modulation (AAIR) 197
right axis deviation 15
    atrial fibrillation with RBBB **134–135**
    chronic lung disease 307, **310–311**
    conduction abnormalities with 89, **92–93**
    first degree block with RBBB **182–183**
    Friedreich's ataxia **344–345**
    hyperkalaemia **330–331**
    in infants 53
    left posterior hemiblock **92–93**
    mitral stenosis and pulmonary
        hypertension **292–293**

normal ECG 15, **16–17**, 55, **306**, 307,
    347
pulmonary embolism 247, **248–249**
pulmonary stenosis **322–323**
right ventricular hypertrophy 305,
    306–307
right ventricular outflow tract tachycardia
    144, **144–145**
right bundle branch block (RBBB)
    acute inferior infarction with **236–237**,
        237
    anterior myocardial infarction with 236,
        236–237
    atrial septal defect **326–327**, 327
    Brugada syndrome *vs* 81
    causes 348
    congenital heart disease **321**, **324–325**,
        325
    first degree block with 89, **90–91**,
        174–175, 175, **182–183**
    healthy people 54
        partial RBBB 25, **26–27**
    inferior myocardial infarction with
        possible anterior ischaemia 237,
        238–239
    investigations 56, **57**
    junctional tachycardia with 135, **136–137**
    left anterior hemiblock and 89, **90–91**,
        92–93
    left anterior hemiblock and first degree
        block with 89, **92–93**
    left anterior hemiblock and second degree
        (2:1) block with 89, **94–95**
    partial 25, **26–27**, **34–35**, **134–135**, 135,
        292–293
        trauma associated **342–343**
    prognosis 54–55
    ventricular extrasystoles with **114–115**
right coronary artery, normal *vs* occluded
    215
right-sided heart disease 303–311
    causes 303
right ventricular hypertrophy 25, **66–67**,
    305–311, **306–307**, **308–309**
    breathlessness and 303, **306–307**,
        308–309
    causes 303
    chest pain and **253**, 307
    ECG features 247, 305, **306**, 307

alternative causes of **306**
    in congenital heart disease **321**, 323,
        324–325
    in infants/young children 52, **52–53**,
        320, **321**
    Fallot's tetralogy **324–325**, 325
    normal variant *vs* 39, **253**
    pattern in pulmonary hypertension 247
    T wave inversion 39, 307, **308–309**
    thromboembolic pulmonary hypertension
        67
right ventricular infarction 228
    acute 228, **228–229**
    inferior infarction with 228, **228–229**
right ventricular outflow tract ventricular
    tachycardia (RVOT-VT) **104–105**,
    105, 144, **144–145**
    management, ablation 162
right ventricular pacemakers (VVI) **189**,
    189–195
    bipolar **190–191**, 191
    chest X-ray **190**
    ECG appearance 191
    functions **189**, 195
    indications for 189, **207**
    intermittent **192–193**, **194–195**
        atrial flutter with **194–195**, 195
    rate response modulation (VVIR) 195
    unipolar 191, **192–193**
R–R interval
    atrial fibrillation **124–125**
    sinus arrhythmia 2, **2**, **2–3**, **112–113**
RS complexes, normal variations 54–55
RSR¹ pattern 25, **26–27**, 135, 347
    Brugada syndrome **80–81**
    pulmonary embolism **250–251**
    R¹ peak higher **134–135**, 135, **136–137**
    RBBB and acute inferior infarction
        236–237, 237
    RBBB and anterior infarction **236–237**,
        237
    variable peaks, ventricular *vs*
        supraventricular tachycardia
        138–139
RSR¹S¹ pattern 25, **26–27**

S

S wave

acute anterolateral infarction with left
axis deviation **222–223**
deep
causes 347
left posterior hemiblock **92–93**
dominant in lead V₄ **20–21**, 21
normal ECG **20–21**, 21
dominant in leads II/III
left axis deviation **86–87**
normal ECG, size 15, **16–17**, **18–19**,
19–25, **24–25**, 25
notched **26–27**
persistent (lead V₆) **10–11**, 307
chronic lung disease **304–305**, 305,
307, **310–311**
mitral stenosis and pulmonary
hypertension **292–293**
pulmonary embolism 247, **248–249**,
310–311, 311
pulmonary stenosis **322–323**
right ventricular and right atrial
hypertrophy **304–305**
R wave size balance 15, 25
size, in chest leads 15, **16–17**, **18–19**,
19–25, **24–25**
'salvo' 152
second degree block **84–85**, 179, **180–181**
2:1 **86–87**, 179, **180–181**
atrial flutter with 117, **118–119**
atrial tachycardia with 117
His bundle electrogram 184, **186**
left anterior hemiblock with 89, **94–95**
left anterior hemiblock and RBBB with
89, **94–95**
3:1 179
4:1 block, atrial flutter with 117,
120–121
causes 184
His bundle electrogram 184, **186**
prognosis 54
syncope due to 170
Wenckebach **84–85**
seizures 60, **61**
sensing, by pacemakers 187, 188
atrial 197, 199
shingles, pain 210
sick sinus syndrome 170, 171–175,
172–173
acquired 177

bradycardia–tachycardia syndrome 171,
175
causes 177
pacing, VVI 189, **207**
sinus bradycardia **170–171**
syncope due to 61, 170, 171
silent atrium 169, 171, 174
single-chamber pacemakers 188, **189**, **207**
sinoatrial disease see sick sinus syndrome
sinoatrial node 82–83
abnormal function 171
inhibition 150, **151**
sinus arrest **173**, 175
sinus arrhythmia 2, 113
healthy people 2, **2–3**, 55
prognosis 55
symptoms with **112–113**, 113
sinus bradycardia 3, **4–5**, 5, 169, **170–171**,
172–173
athletes **4–5**, 5, 49
causes 5, **337**
investigations 57
sinus pauses 171, **172**
sinus rhythm 2, **2**, 127
irregular see sinus arrhythmia
symptoms with **112–113**, 113
syncope causes associated 61
WPW syndrome **108–109**
sinus tachycardia 3, **4–5**, 59, **112–113**
causes 3, 113
diagnosis from symptoms 59, **59**
healthy people 3, **4–5**
investigations 57
management 154
palpitations due to 59, 113, 152
paroxysmal tachycardia vs 59, **59**
pulmonary embolism **246–247**
sodium channels, abnormal, Brugada
syndrome 81
Sokolov-Lyon voltage criterion 295
sotalol, torsade de pointes due to 146
spasm, coronary arteries 247
spinal pain 210
ST segment 31
chest pain diagnosis, pitfalls 256–257,
258–259, **260–261**, **262–263**
depression
anterior ischaemia **242–243**, 243,
244–245

digoxin causing 31, 257, **262–263**,
334–335, 335
exercise test discontinuation 271
exercise testing **272–273**, 273, **278–279**
horizontal, in ischaemia 31, 34, 241,
272–273
nonspecific 31, 35, **36–37**
normal ECG 31, **34–35**, 35, **36–37**
posterior infarction **226–227**, 227
pregnancy 55
supraventricular tachycardia, ischaemia
and **106–107**
unstable angina 213
see also NSTEMI
downward-sloping
digoxin causing 257, **262–263**,
334–335, 335, **336–337**
raised, Brugada syndrome **80–81**
ECG interpretation pitfalls 256–257,
258–259, **260–261**, **262–263**
elevation 31, **32–33**, 214
acute anterior and old inferior
infarction 231, **232–233**
acute inferior infarction **214–215**, 215,
230–231
acute lateral infarction 217, **220–221**
anterior infarction **218–219**
arched, 'early repolarization' 31, **42–43**
causes 35
exercise testing **274–275**, 275
inferior and right ventricular infarction
228, **228–229**
multiple infarctions **230–231**, 231,
232–233
myocardial infarction (STEMI) 31,
213, 214–240, 264
normal ECG 31, **32–33**
pericarditis **250–251**, 251
persistent 225
posterior infarction **226–227**, 227
high take-off 31, **32–33**, 252, **260–261**
isoelectric **30–31**, 31
nonspecific changes in myocardial
infarction **210–211**
normal exercise testing **272–273**
normal variations 31, **32–35**, **36–37**, 55
upward-sloping **30–31**, 31, 273, **278–279**
STEMI 31, 213, 214–240, 264
acute inferior **214–215**, 215

anterior NSTEMI with 231, **232–233**
acute lateral 217, **220–221**
anterior 217
definition/criteria 213
lateral 217, **222–223**
management 285
NSTEMI *vs* 241, 264
old anterior infarction **224–225**, 225
sequence of features characteristic of 213,
  214–215, 264
sternum, depression 21
Stokes–Adams attack **61**, 179, **182–183**
stress echocardiography **268–269**
stress MRI **268–269**
subarachnoid haemorrhage 253, **344–345**,
  345
subendocardial infarction 241
sudden death **61**
  coronary disease 213
  long QT syndrome and 76, 77
  ventricular fibrillation causing **100**
supraventricular extrasystoles **6–7**, 7, 55,
  114–115, 115
  management 152
  normal people **6–7**, 7, 55
  ventricular extrasystoles *vs* **114–115**
supraventricular rhythms 117, 135
supraventricular tachycardia **106–107**, 117,
  126
  ambulatory ECG 96, 150
  arising in AV node, focal junctional
    tachycardia 102
  broad complex tachycardia 126–127,
    136–137
  causes 152
  ECG criteria 127
  palpitations due to 152
  terminology 117
  ventricular tachycardia *vs* 135, **136–137**,
    138–139
  WPW syndrome similarities 107,
    147–149
syncope 59, 60
  cardiovascular causes **61**, 64–69
  aortic stenosis 64, **64–65**, **65**
  arrhythmias 61, **61**
  hypertrophic cardiomyopathy 67,
    68–69
  mitral stenosis 69

pulmonary emboli 67
carotid sinus hypersensitivity 150
definition/meaning 60
diagnosis of causes **61**, 64, 67
ECG features between attacks 64–95, **65**,
  96
long QT syndrome causing 76–77
neurally-mediated syndromes **61**
physical examination 64, 103
pre-excitation syndromes causing 69
quinidine 341
second degree block and 170
sick sinus syndrome 61, 170, 171
tachycardia 69–81
  ECG between attacks 69–81
Syndrome X 277
systemic diseases, ECG in 327, 329
systolic pressure, exercise testing
  discontinuation 271

T

T wave 37–45, 247
abnormalities, investigations **57**
biphasic **34–35**, **52–53**
  in V₃ **40–41**
chest pain diagnosis, pitfalls **256–257**,
  258–259, **260–261**, **262–263**
flat, hypokalaemia **334–335**, 335
flattening, nonspecific **44–45**, 45,
  210–211, 257, **262–263**
inversion 39, 45, 256
  abnormal, prevalence 54
  acute inferior (STEMI) and anterior
    (NSTEMI) infarction 231,
    232–233
  amiodarone causing **338–339**
  anorexia nervosa **342–343**
  anterior 252, 256
  anterior NSTEMI **240–241**, 241
  anxiety associated 45
  black people 39, **42–43**, 252, **306**, 307,
    347
  causes 39, **306**, 307
  digoxin effect 257, **262–263**
  dominant R wave (V₁) with, normal
    variant 307, **308–309**
  hypertrophic cardiomyopathy 67,
    68–69, 299, **300–301**

inferior infarction **140–141**, **214–215**,
  216–217
ischaemia 257 307, **298–299**, 299
lateral 256, 257, **258–259**, 295, 297,
  299
lateral infarction **222–223**
in lead III 37, **38–39**, 39, **210–211**
left anterior hemiblock 299, **302–303**
left bundle branch block **66–67**
left ventricular hypertrophy **64–65**,
  252–253, **253**, 256, **260–261**,
  292–293, **296–297**, 297
left ventricular hypertrophy *vs*
  ischaemia **298–299**, 299,
  300–301
left ventricular strain 297
long QT interval and 256, **258–259**
NSTEMI 213, 241, 246
pulmonary embolism 39, **246–247**,
  247, **248–249**
pulmonary stenosis **322–323**
right ventricular hypertrophy **66–67**,
  305, 307, **308–309**
second degree block **84–85**
supraventricular extrasystoles
  114–115
trauma associated **342–343**
unexplained T wave abnormality with
  256, **258–259**
upright on exercise
  (pseudonormalization) 275,
  276–277
in VL, athletes **50–51**
in VL, left anterior hemiblock **88–89**
voltage criteria with **294–295**, 295,
  297
in VR **36–37**, 37
in VR, V₁-V₂ 39, **40–41**, **42–43**
WPW syndrome, type A **70–71**
WPW syndrome, type B **74–75**,
  258–259
hypertrophic cardiomyopathy 299
left anterior hemiblock 299
nonspecific changes in myocardial
  infarction **210–211**
normal variations 39, 45, 54–55
peaked 347
  hyperkalaemia **330–331**, 331,
    332–333

normal ECG **12–13**, **44–45**, 45, **332–333**, 333
in prolonged QT syndrome due to amiodarone **78–79**
unexplained abnormality 256, **258–259**
ventricular extrasystoles 115
tachycardia 102–167
antidromic reciprocating 106–107, **108**, 147
atrial *see* atrial tachycardia
atrioventricular nodal reciprocating 109
AV nodal re-entry *see* atrioventricular nodal re-entry tachycardia (AVNRT)
carotid sinus pressure 152
enhanced automaticity *vs* re-entry 111
exercise-induced 144
fascicular 135, **136–137**
junctional *see* atrioventricular nodal re-entry tachycardia (AVNRT)
management 152, 154–155
ICD 167
mechanisms 102–111
enhanced automaticity and triggered activity 102–105
re-entry causing arrhythmias 105–111, **107**
re-entry mechanisms 69, 102, 106
non-paroxysmal 102
orthodromic 106, 123
orthodromic reciprocating 106, **108**
pacemaker-mediated 203, **205**
palpitations and syncope symptoms 69–81
paroxysmal 59, **59**
reciprocating 106
right ventricular outflow tract 144, **144–145**
symptomatic 113–149
extrasystoles causing 115
sinus rhythm with 113
ventricular tachycardia forms 144–146
WPW syndrome association 147–149
syncope due to **61**
in WPW syndrome 72, 106–107, **108**
third degree block *see* complete (third degree) block
thromboembolic pulmonary hypertension 67, 247

thyrotoxicosis **326–327**, 327
Tietze's syndrome 211
tilt testing 150
torsade de pointes ventricular tachycardia 76, **76**, 77, 144, 146, **146**, **147**
transition point 19, **20–21**, 21, 307
right ventricular hypertrophy 305
shift, pulmonary embolism 247
trauma, abnormal ECG **342–343**, 343
treadmill, exercise testing 270
tricuspid stenosis **304–305**, 305
trifascicular block 89, **92–93**
'triggered activity' 102–105
ablation therapy 157
cause 105
troponin, elevation 212, 241, 264
causes (not myocardial infarction) 212
in myocardial infarction 212, 213, 264

U

U wave 47
anorexia nervosa **342–343**
hypokalaemia 47, **334–335**, 335
normal ECG **46–47**, 47, 55
athletes **50–51**

V

valve disease 288
vasovagal attack 5, 61, 169
ventricular aneurysm 225
ventricular escape beat **83**
ventricular extrasystoles **6–7**, 7, 96, **114–115**, 115
exercise-induced 282, **284**
investigations 56, **57**
management 152
normal ECGs **6–7**, 7
pregnancy 52, 54
prevalence 54
prognosis 55
R on T phenomenon 115, **116**, **162–163**
RBBB with **114–115**
supraventricular extrasystoles *vs* **114–115**
ventricular fibrillation 162, **162–163**
exercise-induced 282, **284**
management 164, **165**

DC conversion **165**
ICD **166**
R on T phenomenon **162–163**
WPW syndrome with atrial fibrillation 149
ventricular hypertrophy
biventricular **321**
see also left ventricular hypertrophy; right ventricular hypertrophy
ventricular pacing 191, **198–199**, 199
ventricular standstill, ambulatory ECG recording **97**
ventricular tachycardia 109, **110**, 126–127, **130**, 131–135, **132–133**, **134–135**
ambulatory ECG recording **96**
broad QRS complexes 126–127, **130**, 131, **132–133**, **134–135**
capture beat 142, **142–143**
catheter ablation 162
causes 126–127, 152
concordance (QRS complexes) 131, **132–133**, **134–135**, 135
digoxin toxicity **336–337**, 337
ECG criteria 127, 131
episodes, in long QT syndrome 77
exercise-induced 144, **151**
fusion beat 142, **142–143**
ICD cardioversion **165**, **166**, 167
management 155
ablation 162
monomorphic 144
myocardial infarction 131, **132–133**
paroxysmal 76, 155
polymorphic **100**, 144, **146**
see also torsade de pointes ventricular tachycardia
prolonged QT syndrome with 76–77
pulseless, management 164
re-entry causing 109, **110**
RVOT-VT *see* right ventricular outflow tract ventricular tachycardia (RVOT-VT)
second R peak 135
special forms, symptomatic patients 144–146
supraventricular tachycardia *vs* 135, **136–137**, **138–139**
torsade de pointes 144, **146**, **147**
'writhing' polymorphic 144, **146**

verapamil 135, 154
voltage criteria, left ventricular hypertrophy **294–295**, 295, 297, 299
VVI pacing *see* right ventricular pacemakers (VVI)

W

'wandering atrial pacemaker' 49
warfarin 154
Wenckebach phenomenon **84–85**
wide-area circumferential ablation (WACA) 158

Wolff–Parkinson–White (WPW) syndrome 69–72, 73, 105, 106, **148–149**, **258–259**
atrial fibrillation with 73, **148–149**, 149
broad complex tachycardia associated 107, 147–149, **148–149**
ECG diagnostic pitfalls **253**
ECG features summary 73
management 155
  ablation 157, 158
prevalence 72
re-entry pathway **105**, 106, 147

sinus rhythm **70–71**, **72–73**, **108–109**
tachycardias 106–107, **108**, 147–149
type A 69–72, **70–71**, 70–73, **108–109**, **148–149**, 255, **256–257**
after cardioversion **108–109**
type B 69–72, **74–75**, **258–259**, 299, **302–303**
  left ventricular hypertrophy *vs* 299, **302–303**

X

X-rays, chest *see* chest X-rays